Simulation and NCSBN Clinical Judgment Measurement Model

A Nurse Educator's Guide to Innovative Program Development

Laura McIlvoy, Ph.D., RN

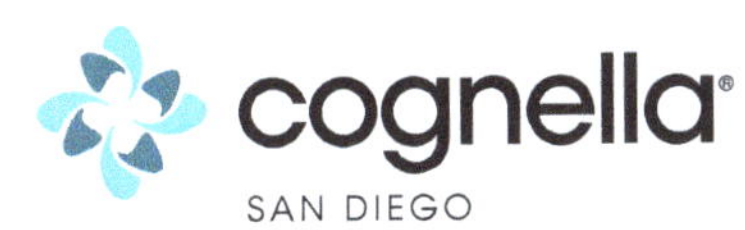

Bassim Hamadeh, CEO and Publisher
Amanda Martin, Executive Publisher
Amy Smith, Associate Editorial Manager
Abbey Hastings, Senior Production Editor
Jess Estrella, Senior Graphic Designer
Kylie Bartolome, Licensing Specialist
Natalie Piccotti, Director of Marketing
Kassie Graves, Senior Vice President, Editorial
Alia Bales, Director, Project Editorial and Production

Printed in the United States of America.

Brief Contents

Contents

Reviewers

Valerie J. Diaz, DNP, CRNA, PMHNP-BC, APRN, CNE, CHSE, CAPT, USN, NC
Department of Nurse Anesthesiology
Nicole Wertheim College of Nursing & Health Sciences
Florida International University

Marisue Rayno, RN, MSN, EdD
Luzerne County Community College

Cynthia Rodriguez-Wewerka, MSN, RN, CNE
Front Range Community College
School of Nursing Sciences

Jennifer Teater, EdD, RN
Indiana University Southeast School of Nursing

CHAPTER 1

Introduction to Mannequin-Based Clinical Simulation Program That Incorporates the CJMM

Learning Outcomes

- Examine the history of mannequin-based clinical simulation.
- Apply a theoretical foundation in developing clinical simulation.
- Evaluate the CJMM and integrate it into educational strategies.
- Recognize the role clinical judgment plays in rescuing patients.
- Incorporate the Healthcare Simulation Standards of Best Practice in all simulation scenarios.

In the Beginning: Clinical Simulation History

As early as the 1800s, models of body parts were used for task training in nursing. By 1910 a full body static mannequin was introduced, and a baby mannequin followed in 1913. By the 1980s computer-assisted instruction (CAI) became part of nursing education modalities. CAI provided information, scenarios, and testing and allowed students to move through the content at their own speed. During this time, a small number of nursing students were fortunate to have access to the early versions of mannequin-based simulation. It wasn't until the early 2000s that mannequin-based simulation became widespread in undergraduate nursing education (Nehring & Lashley, 2009).

Computer-Controlled Mannequin Simulation

In the mid-1960s an engineer along with a physician built the first computer-controlled simulation of the whole patient mannequin, SIMONE, to fulfill the need to develop peacetime applications for training anesthesia residents that "posed significantly less threat to patient safety" (Cooper & Taqueti, p 112). Only one was developed, as the demand for its use was nonexistent. In the late 1960s Dr. Michael Gordon introduced a cardiology patient simulator named Harvey. This model survived to undergo many upgrades and is now available as Next Generation Harvey via Laerdal Simulation. During the 1980s multiple cardiac, anesthesia, and surgical procedure mannequins were developed for resident and nursing student training. Interestingly, key funding for surgical procedure mannequins was provided by the Defense Advancement Research Project Agency (DARPA). During the 1980s and 1990s, high-tech simulation mannequins primarily used in anesthesia training appeared. In 1992 the CASE system was developed at Stanford and incorporated the training curriculum Anesthesia Crisis Resource Management where critical events were introduced in an effort to produce subject response. The success of this type of patient scenario produced simulation moving into an educational model. As subjects were observed and outcomes measured, performance assessment included student behavior skills. In addition, debriefing via watching videotapes of simulation scenarios occurred for the first time (Cooper & Taqueti, 2004). Concurrently, the 1960 Resusci Anne, developed by Asmund Laerdal, slowly morphed into the SimMan in the 1990s.

Mannequin Fidelity

Mannequins (also referred to as *manikins* or *patient simulators*) have either low, moderate, or high fidelity. *Fidelity* refers to the level of reality the mannequin brings to a simulation. A *low-fidelity simulator*, frequently referred to as a *skills trainer*, is a basic mannequin that is not computer controlled. It is a full-body mannequin with realistic anatomical parts that facilitates education and practice of basic nursing skills such as hygiene with linen change, intravenous fluid and medication administration, dressing changes, any kind of ostomy care, and the insertion of urinary and gastric tubes. A *medium-fidelity simulator* is computer controlled, frequently via a handheld device, and usually has all the advantages of a low-fidelity mannequin with the addition of the sound of breathing with no chest rise, manual blood pressure readings, and the auscultation of heart/breath sounds. *High-fidelity simulators* are computer-controlled mannequins that react physiologically as a real person would. They have breathing with chest rise, can be intubated and placed on a ventilator, and have pupils that constrict and dilate and eyes that follow a person around the room. They can be programmed to react appropriately to medications, have conversations with a nurse, experience a seizure, and respond the same way a person would to anything a student does to them. The cost of these high-fidelity patient simulators is generally $60,000 to $100,000 depending on the costs of additional abilities, monitors, and warranties. Any of these mannequins can be connected to a computer-controlled bedside monitor that displays vital signs such as heart rate, respiratory rate, blood pressure, temperature, and, in the case of a high-fidelity mannequin, the advanced cardiac measurements that a pulmonary artery catheter would produce.

Theoretical Foundations That Guide Mannequin-Based Simulation

In 2005, Dr. Pamela Jeffries, working with the National League for Nursing (NLN), developed the NLN Jeffries simulation framework, which incorporated the following components: teacher, student, educational practices, simulation design characteristics, and outcomes (see Figure 1.1). Each component of the framework is associated with variables. These components are linked to associated variables that provide context for the framework. The teacher/student variables are basic attributes of both components. The educational practices

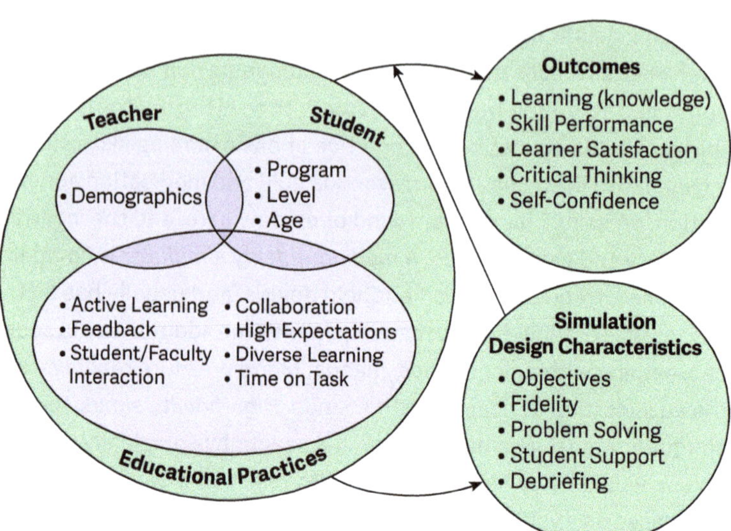

FIGURE 1.1 NLN Jeffries Simulation Framework

component incorporates best practice variables of teaching such as active learning, feedback, student–faculty interactions, and high expectations. These three components connect to both the simulation design characteristics and outcomes. The simulation design characteristics utilize variables that are essential for a simulation experience to be an effective learning environment. The outcomes variables are the desired results students should gain from the simulation experience (Jeffries, 2005).

In 2015 this framework evolved into the NLN Jeffries simulation theory (Jeffries et al., 2015; see Figure 1.2). The background includes goals and specific expectations of the simulation as well as how the simulation fits within the larger curriculum. The time and resources needed are also considered part of the background. The design incorporates the specific learning objectives for each simulation scenario that in turn guide the content, problem-solving activities, equipment and moulage used, student and facilitator responses, and debriefing strategies.

The actual simulation experience requires an environment that is experiential, interactive, collaborative, and learner-centered and

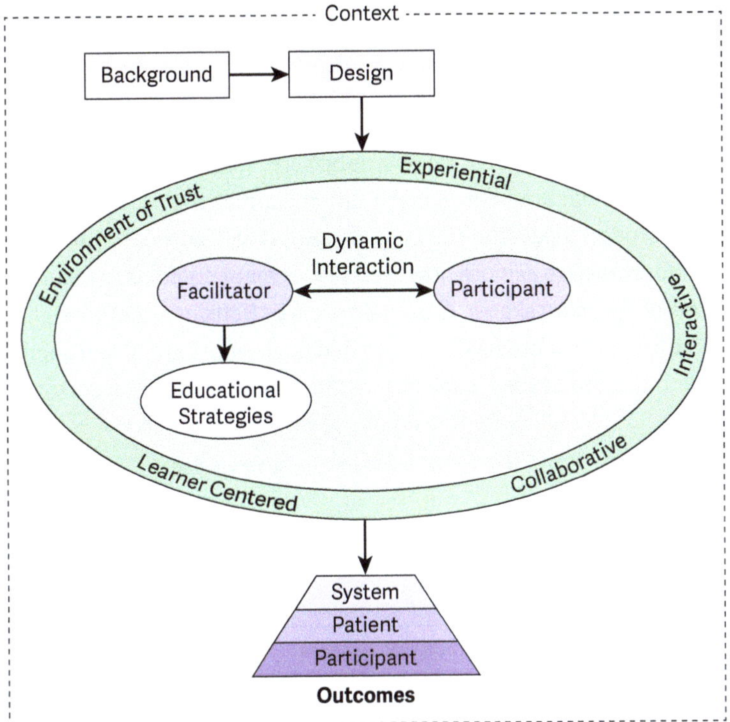

FIGURE 1.2 NLN Jeffries Simulation Theory

establishes an environment of trust. The background influences the design by achieving the goals and specific expectations for the scenario. The design includes the specific learning objectives of the scenario, progression of the activities within the scenario, and participant and observer roles. The facilitator's skill, educational techniques, preparation, and experience affect the simulation experience, as does the relationship between the facilitator and the participant. The age, gender, level of anxiety, self-confidence, and preparation, and skill level of the participant impact the learning experience.

Outcomes are divided into three parts: system, patient, and participant. The participant outcomes are the focus of the literature, specifically the outcomes of satisfaction, self-confidence, learning, and behavior. Literature on patients and systems is emerging (Jeffries et al., 2015).

National Council of State Boards of Nursing Clinical Judgment Measurement Model (CJMM)

The National Council of State Boards of Nursing's (NCSBN, 2019) Clinical Judgment Measurement Model (CJMM) clarifies the process through which students develop clinical judgment (see Figure 1.3). This model was developed to explore how clinical judgment could be measured in terms of licensure exams. A journal article by Betts et al. (2019) explains that the CJMM contains four layers that begin with Layer 0 and become interconnected as the model progresses. Layer 0 represents recognition

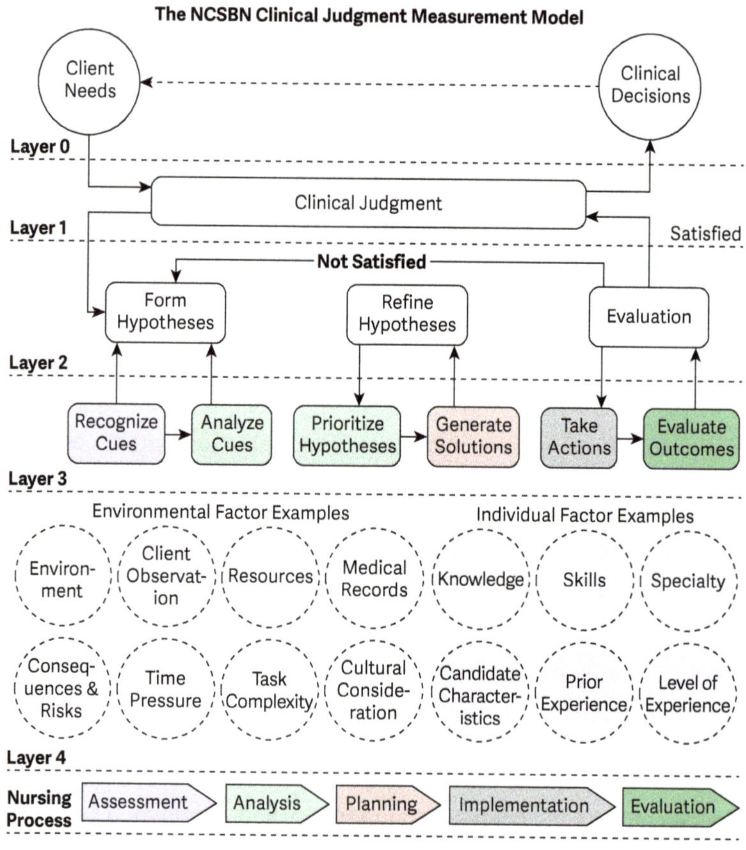

FIGURE 1.3 CJMM

of client needs and connects them to clinical decisions. Layers 1, 2, and 3 delineate the cognitive process of how nurses make clinical judgments using a feedback loop. Layer 3 includes six actions:

1. Recognize cues.
2. Analyze cues.
3. Prioritize hypotheses.
4. Generate solutions.
5. Take actions.
6. Evaluate outcomes.

Within these three layers, hypotheses can be developed and validated or discarded depending on the connection made by recognizing specific cues. The Level 3 actions are measurable and outline how nurses assess cues to generate solutions that lead to treatment solutions. These actions are evaluated for improved outcomes. All of these steps that loop back and forth using clinical judgment result in clinical decisions and flow back to Layer 0, client needs. Layer 4 incorporates environmental and individual factors that could possibly impact the process of clinical judgment (Betts et al., 2019).

The five steps of the nursing process can be found within the CJMM: assessment (cues), diagnosis (generate solutions), planning (hypotheses, solutions), implementation (take actions), and evaluation (evaluate outcomes). Both models provide a process through which nurses can determine what is happening with their patient, consider priorities, take actions, and evaluate outcomes. The CJMM focuses on an algorithm type of thinking that provides for early recognition and an assessment plan that continues until a correct hypothesis is developed to provide appropriate action. It also teaches a level of autonomy to nurses that could improve the timeliness of interventions that will result in saving the patient.

Organized programs of clinical simulation that flow from entry-level students to senior students can provide the process through which students acquire the cognitive, psychomotor, and affective skills necessary to acquire clinical judgment. This book will provide faculty with the details of the process of setting up such a program by providing an in-depth description of how to redesign a fundamentals course into clinical simulation, the importance of performing a program and course needs assessment, and how to take the results of the needs assessment and create simulation objectives for your program and selected courses. Designing a specific scenario that is driven by these objectives and includes measurable student performance behaviors (SPBs) based on the CJMM (specifically, Layer 3) will be explained with examples of SPBs and simulation scenarios. The measurement of SPBs will provide assessment data that is longitudinal, assesses retention of learning, and calculates the success of the CJMM inclusion in providing clinical judgment readiness. How to calculate and use this assessment data will be discussed.

Organizations That Support Clinical Simulation

The International Nursing Association for Clinical Simulation and Learning (INACSL) is an association with over 3,000 members that is "dedicated to advancing the science of healthcare simulation" (About section, n.d.–a). It began with a group of nursing educators meeting in 1976, who continued to grow the idea until 2001 when they decided to create an organization, named it INACSL in 2002, and incorporated it in 2003. *Clinical Simulation in Nursing* is the official journal of INACSL and is a benefit of membership. The journal is published monthly with articles on these selected topics (Nursingsimulation.org, n.d.):

- research articles and literature reviews about simulation
- innovative teaching/learning strategies using simulation
- updates on guidelines, regulations, and legislative policies that impact simulation
- leadership for simulation
- simulation operations
- clinical and academic uses of simulation

INACSL sponsors a 4-day convention every summer that has a program focused on simulation with national simulation experts speaking and many poster presentations that cover a variety of simulation topics. Membership in INACSL includes a discounted price on registration.

The Society for Simulation in Healthcare (SSH) was established in 2004 and represents an interprofessional membership focused on improving the quality of healthcare. They offer four simulation certifications: CHSE (Certified Healthcare Simulation Educator), CHSE-A (Certified Healthcare Simulation Educator-Advanced), CHSOS (Certified Healthcare Simulation Operator Specialist), and CHSOS-A (Certified Healthcare Simulation Operator Specialist-Advanced). Their journal, *Simulation in Healthcare,* is multidisciplinary and publishes articles relevant to simulation technology, simulation centers, and the development of educational and competency standards. The SSH sponsors an annual conference, The International Meeting on Simulation Healthcare (IMSH) that offers hundreds of presentations that provide tools, resources, and industry aimed at impacting delivery systems and practice.

Healthcare Simulation Standards of Best Practice

In 2021 the INACSL Standards Committee introduced the fourth edition of the Healthcare Simulation Standards of Best Practice (HSSOBP; INACSL Standards Committee, 2021a). These evidence-based standards provide a detailed process that faculty can use to design, implement, and evaluate simulation-based experiences. There are 10 standards outlined by the INACSL (n.d.-b):

- Professional development
- Prebriefing
- Simulation design
- Facilitation
- The debriefing process
- Operations
- Outcomes and objectives
- Professional integrity
- Simulation-enhanced interprofessional education
- Evaluation of learning and performance

How to ensure that these standards are incorporated into your simulation operation will be covered throughout this book.

Simulation Glossary

The INACSL Standards Committee (2021b) developed the *Healthcare Simulation Standards of Best Practice Simulation Glossary*. All the simulation terms used in this book can be found within the glossary or defined within the text of this book.

The Agency for Healthcare Research and Quality partnered with the Society for Simulation in Healthcare to develop the *Healthcare Simulation Dictionary* (2nd ed.; Lioce et al., 2020), which includes 170 definitions of healthcare simulation terms. A pdf of the dictionary is available online (https://www.ahrq.gov/sites/default/files/wysiwyg/patient-safety/resources/simulation/sim-dictionary-2nd.pdf).

Clinical Simulation

A simple definition of *clinical simulation* is that it is an active learning method that is a technique, not a technology, involving environments that are reality-based where students are guided during an immersive simulated clinical experience and allowed to gain the knowledge and skills required of nurses in a safe environment (Lateef, 2010). As medical errors are the third leading cause of death in the United States, healthcare must strive to find modalities that help nursing students acquire the required clinical judgment necessary to prevent errors and intervene in time to rescue their patients.

Failure to rescue (*FTR*) is a failure or delay in recognizing and responding to a hospitalized patient experiencing complications from a disease process or medical/nursing intervention (Hall et al., 2020). Nurses are at the bedside and can recognize and act on warning signs of patient deterioration. Rescuing patients requires nurses who have the clinical judgment to recognize these warning signs and to promptly communicate them to the healthcare provider. The current nursing shortage is negatively impacted by new nurses who do not possess the skill of clinical judgment and thereby are unable to recognize the early signs of patient deterioration (Jessee, 2021). The CJMM describes how nurses acquire clinical judgment over time. The transfer-appropriate processing model asserts that learning occurs when information is retrieved using the same process that was used to acquire it (Morris et al., 1977). Therefore, learning that occurs during clinical simulations that are realistic and focused on clinical judgment is more likely to be retrieved later in a real-life clinical situation that requires clinical judgment. This theory necessitates that simulation scenarios be based on the environment and flow of events that reproduce the emergent situation. This cannot be achieved in a 20- to 30-minute scenario. Scenarios need to replicate the situation, which would take 45 to 90 minutes, or be even longer to account for the increased time it would take for students to problem solve. This is why using a team of students in this kind of scenario provides a mechanism for the team to problem solve among themselves while experiencing team dynamics.

Summary

Clinical simulation is the ideal active learning strategy for nursing education. There are many resources available that help in the design of an exceptional simulation program. Using a theoretical foundation, incorporating standards of best practice, and using the clinical judgment model are all necessary introductory steps. As this book progresses, the specifics of producing an organized program of clinical simulation that incorporates these steps and supports student acquisition of clinical judgment will be provided.

References

Betts, J., Muntean, W., Kim, D., Jorion, N., & Dickison, P. (2019). Building a method for writing clinical judgment items for entry-level nursing exams. *Journal of Applied Testing Technology, 20*(Suppl. 2), 21–36.

Cooper, J. B., & Taqueti, V. R. (2004). A brief history of the development of mannequin simulators for clinical education and training. *Quality and Safety in Health Care,* 2004(Suppl 1). i11–i18. doi: 10.1136/qshc.2004.009886

Hall, K. K., Lim, A., & Gale, B. (2020). Failure to rescue. In K. K. Hall, S. Shoemaker-Hunt, L. Hoffman et al. (Eds.). *Making healthcare safer III: A critical analysis of existing and emerging patient safety practices (pp. 2.1–2.16).* Agency for Healthcare Research and Quality. https://www.ncbi.nlm.nih.gov/books/NBK555513

INACSL Standards Committee. (2021a). Healthcare Simulation Standards of Best Practice Professional Development. *Clinical Simulation in Nursing, 58, 5–8. https://doi.org/10.1016/j.ecns.2021.08.007*

Dickison, P., Haerling, K. A., & Lasater, K. (2019). Integrating the National Council of State Boards of Nursing Clinical Judgment Model Into Nursing Educational Frameworks. *Journal of Nursing Education*, 58, 72–78.

INACSL Standards Committee. (2021b). Healthcare Simulation Standards of Best Practice Simulation Glossary. *Clinical Simulation in Nursing, 58*, 57–65. https://doi.org/10.1016/j.ecns.2021.08.017

International Nursing Association for Clinical Simulation and Learning. (n.d.-a). *About INACSL*. Retrieved June 24, 2024, from https://www.inacsl.org/about-inacsl

International Nursing Association for Clinical Simulation and Learning. (n.d.-b). *INACSL Healthcare Simulation Standards of Best Practice with the Support and Input of the Global Community.* Retrieved June 10, 2024, from https://www.inacsl.org/healthcare-simulation-standards

Jeffries, P. R. (2005). A framework for designing, implementing, and evaluating simulations used as teaching strategies in nursing. *Nursing Education Perspectives, 26*(2), 96–103.

Jeffries, P. R. (2021). *The NLN Jeffries Simulation Theory* (2nd ed.). National League of Nursing.

Jeffries, P. R., Rodgers, B., & Adamson K. (2015). NLN Jeffries simulation theory: Brief narrative description. *Nursing Education Perspectives, 36*(5), 292–293.

Jessee, M. A. (2021). An update on clinical judgment in nursing and implications for education, practice, and regulation. *Journal of Nursing Regulation, 12*(3), 50–58.

Lateef, F. (2010). Simulation-based learning: Just like the real thing. *Journal of Emergencies, Trauma, and Shock, 3*(4), 348–352.

Lioce, I., Lopreiato, J., Downing, D., Chang, T. P., Robertson, J. M., Anderson, M., Diaz, D. A., & Spain, A. E. (Eds.). (2020). *Healthcare simulation dictionary* (2nd ed.). Agency for Healthcare Research and Quality.

Morris, C. D., Bransford, J. C., & Franks, J. J. (1977). Levels of processing versus transfer appropriate processing. *Journal of Verbal Learning and Verbal Behavior, 16*(5), 519–533. https://doi.org/10.1016/S0022-5371(77)80016-9

National Council of State Boards of Nursing. (2019). *Clinical Judgment Measurement Model: A framework to measure clinical judgment and decision making.* https://www.nclex.com/Clinical-Judgment-Measurement-Model.page

Nehring, W., & Lashley, R. (2009). Nursing simulation: A review of the past 40 years. *Simulation & Gaming, 40*, 528–552.

Nursingsimulation.org. (n.d.). *Homepage*. Retrieved June 09, 2024, from https://www.nursingsimulation.org/

Society for Simulation in Healthcare. (n.d.). *Homepage*. Retrieved June 09, 2024, from https://www.ssih.org/

Credits

Fig. 1.1: Pamela R. Jeffries and Kristen J. Rogers, "Theorectial Framework for Simulation Design," Simulation in Nursing Education: From Conceptualization to Evaluation, ed. Pamela R Jeffries, p. 23. Copyright © 2007 by National League for Nursing.

Fig. 1.2: Copyright © 2015 by National League for Nursing.

Fig. 1.3: NCSBN, "The NCSBN Clinical Judgment Measurement Model," https://nclex.com/Clinical-Judgment-Measurement-Model.page. Copyright © 2019 by The National Council of State Boards of Nursing (NCSBN).

CHAPTER 2

Introducing Psychomotor Skills Acquisition Using Simulation and the Theory of Deliberate Practice

Learning Outcomes

- Apply the methodology of the deliberate practice theory.
- Recognize the value of using simulation as a technique to teach fundamental skills.
- Plan an innovative simulation experience that incorporates deliberate practice in mastering fundamental nursing skills.

The National Council of State Boards of Nursing's Clinical Judgment Measurement Model (CJMM) provides a method for measuring and deriving correct conclusions that form the clinical judgment and decision-making ability of prospective entry-level nurses. The first step in developing a simulation program based on the CJMM is to remodel the fundamental psychomotor skills course into a simulation experience, as the action level of clinical judgment frequently requires satisfactory skill performance.

First-year nursing students are generally introduced to common psychomotor nursing skills using a variety of educational techniques. Most courses combine a didactic experience with a hands-on lab and possibly a clinical experience. Some nursing students learn a skill once a week and do a check-off of that skill, then perform that skill in clinical. A mechanism for ensuring and measuring retention of learning of psychomotor skills throughout a program is not common. In a clinical setting, students who are unsure of their ability to competently perform psychomotor skills will experience anxiety that focuses their attention on completing the skill and not the bigger picture of using clinical judgment to rescue their patient. This chapter explores how to redesign a nursing fundamentals course that includes reinforcement of learning methods using the theory of deliberate practice in a simulation setting and how these methods can be continued throughout the simulation program.

Deliberate Practice

Deliberate practice is deliberate learning (Clapper & Kardong-Edgren, 2012). It involves practicing a skill under supervision and receiving a debriefing of the skill performance by experienced faculty. This is done repeatedly over time until the student demonstrates mastery (Ericsson, 2008). This requires a template that is evidence-based and does not include "tips" on how to perform the skill. There can only be one way to teach it that everyone employs. Deliberate practice has been used in other fields but only sporadically in nursing. It is most beneficial when it is used throughout a simulation program, as the repetition of skills used in simulated scenarios promotes improved retention of learning (Johnson et al., 2020).

Using Student Simulation Competencies in Program Assessment

As part of a program assessment of student learning for a midwestern school of nursing's simulation program student performance behaviors (SPBs) were developed for every simulation scenario. The program assessment used student success or failure in the performance of these SPBs as senior-level competencies. This was possible because the data was collected during the critical care simulation that occurred 5 months before graduation. Many of the SPBs measured the student performance of psychomotor skills. These types of skills were taught and supposedly mastered as part of the sophomore-level fundamentals course. Data collection began in 2010 as this was when the first group of senior students completed all 3 years of simulation and clinicals in the program. The program assessment data that was collected is presented in Table 2.1 (Mcilvoy & McMahan, 2017, poster presentation).

Gap Analysis

The pass rate for the school of nursing was 75%; therefore, the simulation program set the pass rate for all SPBs at 75%. The first look at the data for successful completion of competencies revealed that many essential skill competencies were performed successfully less than 75% of the time. A *gap analysis* reveals what you have compared to what you should have in terms of knowledge/performance of psychomotor skills (Fater, 2013). In this instance, gap analysis refers to the deficiency in the performance of psychomotor skill competencies compared to the ideal performance (>75%). SPB data was collected for 3 years (2010–2012), revealing unsatisfactory student behaviors in successful completion of psychomotor skills as demonstrated in Table 2.1, data from Before Course Redesign.

Retention of Learning

In response to this gap in performance proficiency, the school of nursing focused on retention of learning. In 2013 the fundamentals course was redesigned into a clinical simulation experience where every lab day occurred in the school simulation hospital (the 12-bed lab). It began with a hospital orientation modeled after how most hospitals orient new nurses. There were two hospital orientation days where the students were introduced to basic hospital psychomotor skills (connecting and priming IV tubing, use of IV pump, glucometer, etc.). The next lab day was admission day, where students admitted their patient, completing all of the necessary admission history paperwork. As they had been taught how to take a patient history and perform a routine physical the semester before, this served as deliberate practice. Hospital Day 1

TABLE 2.1 Senior-Level SPBs Psychomotor Proficiency Before and After Participating in New Fundamentals Course as a Simulation Experience

Senior SPBs BEFORE COURSE REDESIGN				Senior SPBs AFTER COURSE REDESIGN			
STUDENT PERFORMANCE BEHAVIORS ***Basic Admission Scenario (SIM 1)***	**2010 10 scenarios**	**2011 18 scenarios**	**2012 12 scenarios**	**2013 12 scenarios**	**2014 12 scenarios**	**2015 14 scenarios**	**2016 12 scenarios**
Check first ID Check second ID	70%	61%	83% 67%	92% 82%	83% 75%	86% 86%	86% 86%
Change Sterile W-D dressing correctly	71%	75%	67%	91.5%	86%	86%	83%
Hang IVPB with back-priming	29%	75%	100%	100%	50%	86%	100%

Senior SPBs BEFORE COURSE REDESIGN				Senior SPBs AFTER COURSE REDESIGN			
STUDENT PERFORMANCE BEHAVIORS ***Complex Critical Care Scenario (SIM 2)***	**2010 15 scenarios**	**2011 11 scenarios**	**2012 12 scenarios**	**2013 12 scenarios**	**2014 12 scenarios**	**2015 14 scenarios**	**2016 12 scenarios**
Check first ID Check second ID	67%	54%	100%	100%	75%	93% 93%	100% 100%
Change Sterile W-D dressing correctly	57%	64%	76%	91.5%	89%	71%	83%
Hang IV drip medication successfully	43%	0%	83%	-	50%	79%	100%

Abbreviations:

ID: Identification — IVPB: Intravenous Piggyback

W-D: Wet to Dry — IV: Intravenous

Source: Mcilvoy & McMahan, 2017, Poster presentation

to Hospital Day 6 followed with provider orders and a medication administration record for each hospital day. If students have taken a pharmacology course before or concurrently, it would allow for retention of learning if the medications given were the same as what was being studied that week in pharmacology. Students cared for the same 2–4 patients throughout the semester, repeating skills that they had already learned while adding a new skill every week. This repetition resulted in improvement in senior student skill performance (Mcilvoy & McMahan, 2017, poster presentation) as demonstrated in Table 2.1 After Course Redesign.

In 2018, the course was redesigned again to completely integrate the theory of deliberate practice using student mastery video creation for specific high-volume, high-risk skills throughout the simulation program. An improvement in retention of learning was again noted, and program assessment competencies were met.

Specifics of a Redesign for a Fundamentals Course Into Clinical Simulation

To use the theory of deliberate practice with psychomotor skills, a simulated hospital setting works best. It can be formulated as a new nurse would be oriented to a new job, as these are essentially new students to the nursing program. Fundamentals courses include didactic and lab, and the concepts of the didactic content can be paired with the equipment and skills in the simulation scenario. Videos for each skill made by faculty or other sources along with a step-by-step written guide of the skill with reading assignments can be used to prepare students before each simulated hospital day. The lab would need to run like a clinical with each group of students and their clinical faculty assigned 2–4 patients. Each lab group would contain the same patients, so there would only be one set of identical paperwork for each group. These patients can be low-fidelity mannequins that do not need bedside monitors. However, they need to be capable of allowing the students to perform a wide variety of skills. This can be done with even the lowest fidelity of mannequins (see Chapter 7). The instructor would choose

TABLE 2.2 Senior-Level SPBs Psychomotor Proficiency Before and After Participating in Simulation Program with Integration of Deliberate Practice Theory

Senior SPBs BEFORE COURSE REDESIGN			Senior SPBs AFTER COURSE REDESIGN		
STUDENT PERFORMANCE BEHAVIORS ***Basic Critical Care Admission Scenario (SIM 1)*** **SENIOR-LEVEL PROGRAM COMPETENCIES**	**2017 12 scenarios**	**2018 11 scenarios**	**2019 12 scenarios**	**2020 12 scenarios**	**2021 14 scenarios**
Check of two methods of ID	83%	70%	92%*	100%*	100%*
Changes sterile Wet-Dry dressing correctly	100%	60%	100% MV	83% MV	100% MV
Hang IVPB with back-priming	100%	60%	67% MV	100% MV	75% MV
Correct IV priming and pump operation	92%	90%	75% MV	66% MV	100% MV
Draws from arterial line correctly	67%	40%	100% MV	100% MV	100% MV
Infuses blood product correctly	92%	50%	100%#	100%#	66%#
Hangs IV drip medication successfully	92%	90%	67%	66%	100%

STUDENT PERFORMANCE BEHAVIORS ***Complex Critical Care Scenario (SIM 2)*** **SENIOR-LEVEL PROGRAM COMPETENCIES**	**2017 12 scenarios**	**2018 10 Scenarios**	**2019 12 Scenarios**	**2020 11 scenarios**	**2021 11 scenarios**
Check of two methods of ID	92%	60%	100%*	100%*	90%*
Changes sterile Wet-Dry dressing correctly	83%	80%	100% MV	100% MV	100% MV
Hang IVPB with back-priming	83%	100%	100% MV	100% MV	95% MV
Correct IV priming and pump operation	92%	70%	74% MV	92% MV	82% MV
Infuses blood product correctly	83%	80%	100%#	92%#	100%#
Hangs IV drip medication successfully	92%	70%	74%	92%	82%

Abbreviations:

ID: Identification IVPB: Intravenous Piggyback

W-D: Wet to Dry IV: Intravenous

Source: Mcilvoy & McMahan,2020, Poster Presentation

MV = Mastery video made by student for this skill during sophomore fundamentals

** = Safety behavior placed on all scenarios in program*

5–7 skills that require student mastery videos. Having half of the mastery videos due at midterms and the rest due at finals seems to work well. The beginning ones should be easier, and the later ones should cover the more difficult skills. For example, priming IV tubing and placing them successfully in an IV pump along with intramuscular (IM) and subcutaneous (SQ) injections would be beginning skills, whereas IV piggyback (IVPB) and wet-dry sterile dressings and urinary catheterization could be the later skills. If by chance these students are enrolled in pharmacology at the same time as fundamentals, each week's medication could be administered in fundamentals clinical to facilitate retention of learning.

To accommodate the continuing issue of lack of faculty, the clinical simulation could be divided in half and run concurrently. For example, if each lab time is 3 hours, then each session would run for 90 minutes. A faculty with 8–10 students in their clinical group would only have 4–5 students at a time for their 2–3 patients (mannequins) with half the class and a second 90 minutes with the rest of the students. This gives each faculty less students at a time in the scenario to enable a closer look at student practice. The group of students not in simulation could be in another room with one faculty practicing the skill of the week or doing something online like a virtual program. After half the time is over, all the students change place, but faculty remains in the same place. The following examples of each simulation day and their components gives a sample of how the fundamentals simulation experience can be scheduled. However, each day should be tailored to the needs of students, faculty, and the program.

Hospital Orientation Day (HOD) 1 and Day 2

These first 2 days will run differently, as you are introducing concepts, equipment, and skills, modeled after a hospital orientation. They can be blended between lecture and lab, there could be stations that groups rotate through, or any other innovative method can be used.

- Didactic Concepts
    - Theory of deliberate practice
    - Safety

  - Infection control
  - Healthcare practitioner orders
  - Charting
  - Health Insurance Portability and Accountability Act (HIPAA)
  - Medication Administration Parts 1 and 2
  - Sterile technique
  - Baseline medication calculation quiz
  - Faculty demonstration of selected skills

- Clinical Simulation Focus
  - Hospital Orientation Day 1 and 2 student performance objectives (below)
  - Donning sterile gloves
    - This is a skill that can be done at the start of every simulation just to allow hand-eye coordination to improve by the end of the semester.
  - IV tubing priming and IV pump function
    - Use both central (triple lumen and peripherally inserted central catheter lines) and peripheral IV lines.
  - Using glucometer
    - There are several methods for making homemade blood that will show as a blood sugar level on a glucometer (see Chapter 7).
  - Medication administration via percutaneous esophagogastrostomy (PEG) tube
    - Having a PEG tube in all the patients allows students to perform medication calculations and administer the correct amounts of pills and liquids using the evidence-based protocol for giving medications via the PEG. All patients in our lab and in simulation have PEG tubes to allow this level of medication administration. PEG tubes are either taped to skin or inserted through the holes some mannequins have in their chest pieces. They are connected to drainage systems hidden under the bed (see Chapter 7).

Examples of Hospital Orientation Day (HOD) 1 and 2 Student Performance Behaviors

HOD 1 With Faculty at Bedside:

- Performs correct hand hygiene
- Dons sterile gloves
- Primes IV tubing and sets IV pump
- Clears flush syringe of air
- Performs glucose monitoring
- Demonstrates use of bladder scanner
- Performs collection of urine sample from the student volunteer who underwent bladder scanner and compares outcomes
- Demonstrates successful log into Medication Dispensing Unit
- Takes a BP using a cuff

HOD 2 With Faculty at Bedside:

- Performs correct hand hygiene

Demonstrates appropriate donning of personal protective equipment (PPE)

  - Gown
  - Mask
  - Goggles
  - Gloves
- Dons sterile gloves
- Primes IV tubing and sets IV pump and clears IV pump volume
- Clears flush syringe of air
- Flush IV sites:
  - Triple lumen
  - Peripherally inserted central catheter (PICC) line
  - Peripheral lines
- Performs glucose monitoring with glucometer per MD order
  - Documents glucose reading
- PEG tubes and medication administration
- Intramuscular (IM) injection practice
- Subcutaneous (SQ) injection practice
- Bed-to-stretcher transfer

Prebriefing: Preparation and Briefing

The 2021 INACSL standards on prebriefing incorporate preparation and briefing (INACSL Standards Committee, 2021). To facilitate students' preparation for each week, they will need didactic preparation information, such as reading assignments, PowerPoint slides, and so on, available at least 3–5 days in advance. To prepare for the simulation scenario, the patient's information, diagnosis, and expected student performance behaviors should also be available weekly prior to simulation. The patients will need charts (paper or electronic) with weekly new provider orders, Medication Administration Records (MARs), and the like. Each psychomotor skill for the simulation requires a step-by-step rubric for students, either from the book or made by faculty, and a video of the skill is also beneficial (see textbox below).

Rubric: Priming IV Tubing and IV Pump Operation Mastery Video

*Must be filmed so that IV tubing is visible during priming

Supplies: Chart, Alaris pump, IV fluids, primary tubing, alcohol pads, 10 mL flush syringe

1. Check order for correct IV fluids.
2. Check for correct patient ID.
3. Perform hand hygiene.
4. Don gloves.
5. Check patency of IV site:
   - Scrub hub of IV site.
   - Remove air from flush syringe.
   - Check the patency of IV site by flushing with normal saline flush.
6. Open primary tubing.
7. Close roller clamp.
8. Spike IV bag.
9. Hang on IV pole.
10. Squeeze drip chamber.

11. Open roller clamp and prime tubing.
12. Ensure there is NO AIR in the tubing after priming.
13. Close roller clamp.
14. Connect tubing to the IV site.
15. Label tubing.
16. Check orders for IV rate.
17. Place tubing into IV pump.
18. Open roller clamp.
19. Turn pump on.
20. Set IV rate.
21. Set volume to be infused (VTBI).
22. Start pump.

*Continue filming until you see dripping in the drip chamber on film with no alarms sounding.

Briefing for the simulation experience entails meeting with all students and reviewing the patient information and the student performance behaviors they will be completing. As this is a learning experience, allowing students to access the rubric and video during the scenario is something students find very helpful.

Admission Day (Preoperative Day)

This is the day the hospital is introduced as well as the 2–4 patients (or as many that work in your situation) that students will care for every week. It is also preoperative day, as it works well that students are completing not only admission paperwork but also the surgery checklist, as the patient will be going to surgery that afternoon. Having postoperative patients, the following week allows for more skills to be introduced.

- Didactic Concepts
    - Medication reconciliation
    - History
    - Systems assessment
    - Hidden terminology in nursing “slang”

  - IV fluids
  - Insulin and sliding scale
  - Preoperative care
  - Surgery checklist
  - Faculty demonstration of selected skills

- Clinical Simulation Focus
  - Donning sterile gloves
  - MD/NP orders
    - This is placed first for the day, as orders drive nursing practice and will help students get organized for their scenario.
  - Medication reconciliation
    - Patients can have a bag of pills with them, a handwritten list, or bottles of pills for students to use for reconciliation.
  - Forms required for scenario
    - Medication Administration Record (MAR)
    - Provider Orders
    - Surgery Checklist
    - Health History Form
    - Medication Reconciliation Form (Example 2.1)
    - Surgery Consent Form signed by MD and patient

Example 2.1 Admission Medication Reconciliation Form

Allergies: ☐ NKA ______________________________

LIST BELOW ALL OF THE PATIENT'S MEDICATIONS PRIOR TO ADMISSION INCLUDING OTC AND HERBAL MEDS

Source of Medication List (check all used):

☐ Patient written medication list

☐ Patient/family statements

☐ Pharmacy prescription containers

☐ Medications

MEDICATION HISTORY RECORDED/VERIFIED BY:

____

Medication Name	**Dose**	**Route**	**Frequency**	**Last Dose Date/Time**

Healthcare Provider Signature: ______________________________

Signature of Patient/Family who provided information:

____

Each day of simulation requires a list of Student Performance Behaviors that are given to students as part of their preparation for the simulation.

Admission Day Student Performance Behaviors

Mr. Garcia: A 64-year-old Hispanic man diagnosed with community-acquired pneumonia, has a PEG.	Mr. Daniels: A 30-year-old European American man fell, suffered a closed fracture of left femur, history of Crohn's disease with a PEG placed 3 years ago.	Mrs. Green: A 76-year-old African American woman undergoing elective right total hip replacement surgery, PEG placement, with a history of type 2 diabetes.
• Safety: Determines 2 methods of patient identification • Acknowledge MD orders • Obtains blood sugar • Obtains health history from family member and performs medication reconciliation • Administers IV fluids using Alaris pump • Assesses and documents accordingly • Completes Time on Task	• Safety: 2 methods of patient identification • Acknowledge MD orders • Obtains blood sugar check • Obtain health history from family member and perform medication reconciliation • Administers IV fluids using Alaris pump • Assesses and documents accordingly • Gives preop bath and bed linen change • Administers preop medications • Completes preop paperwork • Completes Time on Task	• Safety: 2 methods of patient identification • Acknowledge MD orders • Obtains blood sugar check • Obtain health history from family member and perform medication reconciliation • Administers IV fluids using Alaris pump • Assesses and documents accordingly • Gives preop bath and bed linen change • Administers preop medications • Completes preop paperwork • Completes Time on Task

The following examples of Hospital Day 1 through Hospital Day 4 didactic and clinical simulation focus, with the applicable student performance behaviors, are listed below.

Hospital Day 1 (Postoperative Day 1) Student Performance Behaviors

Mr. Garcia: A 64-year-old Hispanic man diagnosed with community-acquired pneumonia, has a PEG.	Mr. Daniels: A 30-year-old European American man who underwent an open reduction internal fixation (ORIF) of left femur, history of Crohn's disease with a PEG placed 3 years ago.	Mrs. Green: A 76-year-old African American woman who underwent an elective total right hip replacement surgery, PEG placement, with a history of type 2 diabetes.
• Safety: Determines 2 methods of patient identification • Acknowledge MD orders • Obtains blood sugar • Gives medications • Administers IV fluids using Alaris pump • Administers IVPB • Transfuses blood product • Place a condom catheter	• Safety: Determines 2 methods of patient identification • Acknowledge MD orders • Obtains blood sugar • Gives medications • Administers IV fluids using Alaris pump • Manages postoperative pain • Empties and measures output of Jackson-Pratt (JP) drain	• Safety: Determines 2 methods of patient identification • Acknowledge MD orders • Obtains blood sugar • Gives medications • Administers IV fluids using Alaris pump • Manages postoperative pain using a patient-controlled anesthesia (PCA) pump

• Assesses and documents accordingly • Completes Time on Task	• Obtains a wound culture • Administers IVPB • Transfuses blood product • Place a condom catheter • Assesses and documents accordingly • Completes Time on Task	• Empties and measures output of Hemovac drain • Administers IVPB • Transfuses blood product • Assesses and documents accordingly • Completes Time on Task

Hospital Day 2

- Didactic Concepts
    - IVPB
    - PCA pump
    - Postoperative drains
    - Blood product infusion and paperwork
    - Faculty demonstration of selected skills
- Clinical Simulation Focus
    - Donning sterile gloves
    - MD/NP orders
    - Blood product infusion
    - Surgical drain management (Hemovac/Jackson-Pratt)

Hospital Day 2 (Postoperative Day 2) Student Performance Behaviors

Mr. Garcia: A 64-year-old Hispanic man diagnosed with community-acquired pneumonia. He received a tracheotomy at the bedside.	Mr. Daniels: A 30-year-old Caucasian man who underwent an ORIF of left femur. He has a history of Crohn's disease with a PEG placed 3 years ago. His wound culture revealed MRSA in his wound. He received a tracheotomy at the bedside.	Mrs. Green: A 76-year-old African American woman who underwent an elective total right hip replacement surgery, with a history of type 2 diabetes. She has a PEG.
• Safety: Determines 2 methods of patient identification • Acknowledge MD orders • Obtains blood sugar • Gives medications • Administers IV fluids using Alaris pump • Administers IVPB • Transfuses blood product • Performs tracheostomy care • Assesses and documents accordingly • Completes Time on Task	• Safety: Determines 2 methods of patient identification • Acknowledge MD orders • Maintains contact Isolation • Obtains blood sugar • Gives medications • Administers IV fluids using Alaris pump • Manages postoperative pain • Empties and measures output of Jackson-Pratt (JP) drain • Administers IVPB	• Safety: Determines 2 methods of patient identification • Acknowledge MD orders • Obtains blood sugar • Gives medications • Administers IV fluids using Alaris pump • Manages postoperative pain using a PCA pump • Empties and measures output of Hemovac drain • Administers IVPB • Transfuses blood product • Assesses and documents accordingly

	• Transfuses blood product • Performs tracheostomy care • Assesses and documents accordingly • Completes Time on Task	• Places a 40% face mask • Infuse fresh frozen plasma (FFP) transfusion • Assess and document accordingly • Completes Time on Task

Hospital Day 3

- Didactic Concepts
  - Airway and oxygenation
- Clinical Simulation Focus
  - Tracheostomy care
  - PCA
  - Medications
  - Blood product infusion
  - Surgical drain management
  - Nasal Cannula/Oxymizer placement
  - Isolation

Hospital Day 3 (Postoperative Day 3) Student Performance Behaviors

Mr. Garcia: A 64-year-old Hispanic man diagnosed with community-acquired pneumonia.	Mr. Daniels: A 30-year-old European American man who underwent an ORIF of left femur. He has a history of Crohn's disease with a PEG placed 3 years ago.	Mrs. Green: A 76-year-old African American woman who underwent an elective total right hip replacement surgery, with a history of type 2 diabetes. She has a PEG. She received a tracheostomy at the bedside.
• Safety: Determines 2 methods of patient identification • Acknowledge MD orders • Obtains blood sugar • Gives medications • Administers IV fluids using Alaris pump • Transfuses blood product • Performs tracheostomy care • Assesses and documents accordingly • Completes Time on Task	• Safety: Determines 2 methods of patient identification • Acknowledge MD orders • Obtains blood sugar • Gives medications • Administers IV fluids using Alaris pump • Manages postoperative pain • Empties and measures output of Jackson-Pratt (JP) drain • Administers IVPB • Transfuses blood product • Performs tracheostomy care • Assesses and documents accordingly • Completes Time on Task	• Safety: Determines 2 methods of patient identification • Acknowledge MD orders • Obtains blood sugar • Gives medications • Administers IV fluids using Alaris pump • Manages postoperative pain using a PCA pump • Empties and measures output of Hemovac drain • Administers IVPB • Transfuses blood product • Performs tracheostomy care • Assesses and documents accordingly • Completes Time on Task

Hospital Day 4

- Didactic Concepts
  - Midterm
- Clinical Simulation Focus
  - Perform all skills previously taught
  - Begin Mastery Video Faculty Checkoffs for selected skills

Verification of Skill Attainment: Mastery Videos

Faculty must decide on which skills are vital for students to master at the beginning level for their program. To verify mastery of each chosen skill, students must produce a "mastery video" of themselves performing each skill. It is easier if half are due around the time of the midterm and the rest due at the end of the course. Other students will film the student performing the skill. Students are extremely proficient at filming videos on their phones, and it would be rare for a problem to occur.

Each master skill requires a rubric and a faculty-made video for students to reference during learning. To ensure that they have truly mastered the skill before they film, all students require permission from their clinical faculty in the form of a ticket that must be presented the day they film. Below is an example of skills selected and the directions on the mastery videos placed in the syllabus.

The six skills for which students will produce a video verifying their mastery of that skill are:

- Priming IV tubing and IV pump operation
- SQ medication calculation and administration
- IM medication calculation and administration
- IVPB administration with back priming
- Wet-dry dressing with sterile technique
- In & out urinary catheterization

> Students will be able to view a mastery video made by faculty for all six of these skills. Students will have a grading rubric for each of the six nursing skills to assist in their effort to master them. Clinical faculty will work with students during the simulation hours to facilitate mastery of each skill. Once the faculty feels the student has mastered a skill, they will issue the student a ticket that enables them to schedule a time to record their mastery video. If any of the videos are submitted after the due date, the student will be assigned a paper on professionalism by their faculty. If a submitted mastery video is determined to be unsatisfactory, a second attempt at making a mastery video will be allowed and must be submitted within 2 weeks after the original due date. **Failure to submit a satisfactory mastery video for each of the six selected skills will result in an Unsatisfactory grade in this course.**

During the COVID-19 pandemic, the IM medication mastery was demonstrated while giving the COVID-19 vaccine in partnership with a local hospital and the county health department, with multiple faculty on site. Many fundamentals courses include some clinical hours. If this is so, faculty observing the student in clinical performing one of the master skills with no assistance could also be used for a skill mastery checkoff.

Hospital Day 4 (Postoperative Day 4) Student Performance Behaviors

Mr. Garcia: A 64-year-old Hispanic man diagnosed with community-acquired pneumonia.	Mr. Daniels: A 30-year-old European American man who underwent an ORIF of left femur. He has a history of Crohn's disease with a PEG placed 3 years ago.	Mrs. Green: A 76-year-old African American woman who underwent an elective total right hip replacement surgery, with a history of type 2 diabetes. She has a PEG. She received a tracheostomy at the bedside.
• Safety: Determines 2 methods of patient identification • Acknowledge MD orders • Obtains blood sugar • Gives medications • Administers IV fluids using Alaris pump • Transfuses blood product • Performs tracheostomy care • Changes dressing over venous stasis ulcer • Assesses and documents accordingly	• Safety: Determines 2 methods of patient identification • Acknowledge MD orders • Obtains blood sugar • Gives medications • Administers IV fluids using Alaris pump • Manages postoperative pain • Performs wet-to-dry sterile dressing change over surgical wound • Administers IVPB • Transfuses blood product	• Safety: Determines 2 methods of patient identification • Acknowledge MD orders • Obtains blood sugar • Gives medications • Administers IV fluids using Alaris pump • Performs wet-to-dry sterile dressing change over surgical wound • Administers IVPB • Transfuses blood product

• Completes Time on Task	• Performs tracheostomy care • Assesses and documents accordingly • Completes Time on Task	• Manages postoperative pain • Performs tracheostomy care • Assess and document accordingly • Completes Time on Task

- Didactic Concepts
  - Skin impairments
  - Braden Scale
  - Dressing types
  - Sterile dressing changes
- Clinical Simulation Focus
  - Blood transfusion
  - Dressing changes

Hospital Day 5 (Postoperative Day 5) Student Performance Behaviors

Mr. Garcia: A 64-year-old Hispanic man diagnosed with community-acquired pneumonia.	Mr. Daniels: A 30-year-old European American man who underwent an ORIF of left femur. He has a history of Crohn's disease with a PEG placed 3 years ago.	Mrs. Green: A 76-year-old African American woman who underwent an elective total right hip replacement surgery, with a history of type 2 diabetes. She has a PEG. She received a tracheostomy at the bedside.
• Safety: Determines 2 methods of patient identification • Acknowledge MD orders • Obtains blood sugar • Gives medications • Administers IV fluids using Alaris pump • Transfuses blood product • Performs tracheostomy care • Changes dressing over venous stasis ulcer • Places Salem Sump to low continuous suction • Assesses and documents accordingly	• Safety: Determines 2 methods of patient identification • Acknowledge MD orders • Obtains blood sugar • Gives medications • Administers IV fluids using Alaris pump • Manages postoperative pain • Performs wet-to-dry sterile dressing change over surgical wound • Administers IVPB • Transfuses blood product • Performs tracheostomy care	• Safety: Determines 2 methods of patient identification • Acknowledge MD orders • Obtains blood sugar • Gives medications • Administers IV fluids using Alaris pump • Performs wet-to-dry sterile dressing change over surgical wound • Administers IVPB • Transfuses blood product • Manages postoperative pain

• Completes Time on Task	• Places small-bore feeding tube and initiates feeding via enteral feeding protocol • Assesses and documents accordingly • Completes Time on Task	• Performs tracheostomy care • Places small-bore feeding tube and initiates feeding via enteral feeding protocol • Assesses and documents accordingly • Completes Time on Task

- Didactic Concepts
  - Nutrition
  - Gastrointestinal tubes
  - Tube feedings
- Clinical Simulation Focus
  - Dressing types
  - Sterile dressing changes
  - Salem Sump Tubes
  - Small-bore feeding tubes
  - Tube feeding via protocol

Hospital Day 6 (Postoperative Day 6) Student Performance Behaviors

Mr. Garcia: A 64-year-old Hispanic man diagnosed with community-acquired pneumonia.	Mr. Daniels: A 30-year-old European American man who underwent an ORIF of left femur. He has a history of Crohn's disease with a PEG placed 3 years ago.	Mrs. Green: A 76-year-old African American woman who underwent an elective total right hip replacement surgery, with a history of type 2 diabetes. She has a PEG. She received a tracheostomy at the bedside.
• Safety: Determines 2 methods of patient identification • Acknowledge MD orders • Obtains blood sugar • Gives medications • Administers IV fluids using Alaris pump • Transfuses blood product • Performs tracheostomy care • Changes dressing over venous stasis ulcer • Converts Salem Sump to tube feeding via protocol after X-ray clears tube placement	• Safety: Determines 2 methods of patient identification • Acknowledge MD orders • Obtains blood sugar • Gives medications • Administers IV fluids using Alaris pump • Manages postoperative pain • Performs wet-to-dry sterile dressing change over surgical wound • Administers IVPB • Transfuses blood product • Performs tracheostomy care	• Safety: Determines 2 methods of patient identification • Acknowledge MD orders • Obtains blood sugar • Gives medications • Administers IV fluids using Alaris pump • Performs wet-to-dry sterile dressing change over surgical wound • Administers IVPB • Transfuses blood product • Manages postoperative pain

• Performs in-out urinary catheterization • Assesses and documents accordingly • Completes Time on Task	• Places small-bore feeding tube and initiates feeding via enteral feeding protocol • Performs in-out urinary catheterization • Assesses and documents accordingly • Completes Time on Task	• Performs tracheostomy care • Places small-bore feeding tube and initiates feeding via enteral feeding protocol • Performs in-out urinary catheterization • Assesses and documents accordingly • Completes Time on Task

- Didactic Concepts
  - Genitourinary system
  - Urinary catheters
  - Urinary catheterization
    - In and out
    - Continuous
  - Catheter-associated urinary tract infection (CAUTI) guidelines
  - Rapid response
- Clinical Simulation Focus
  - Dressing types
  - Sterile dressing changes
  - Salem Sump Tubes
  - Small-bore feeding tubes
  - Tube feeding via protocol (see Example 2.2)
  - Intermittent urinary catheterization

Example 2.2. Enteral Tube Feeding Protocol

Allergies: ______________________________

Date and Time	WRITTEN ORDERS
	1. Dietary consult
	2. Insert enteral feeding tube 3. Chest X-ray to check placement of feeding tube DO NOT BEGIN FEEDS UNTIL PHYSICIAN VERIFIES TUBE PLACEMENT ☐ Check when physician verification is completed
	4. Continuous tube feeding a. Start type of tube feeding as ordered by physician/dietitian b. Begin at 25 mL/hr continuous feeding using the tube feeding formula ordered by physician c. Advance by 25 mL every 8 hours until 75 mL/hr is reached d. Check tube feeding residual every 4 hours; if greater than 350 mL, replace residual and call physician (do not stop tube feeding) e. Start blood sugar checks every 8 hours and treat high blood sugars as ordered
	5. Bolus tube feeding a. Administer formula and amount order by physician b. Flush tube with 30 mL water before and after bolus feeding
	6. Head of bed elevated at least 45 degrees during feeding
	7. DO NOT hold tube feeding without order from physician
	8. BMP every 3 days, CMP every 7 days while tube feeding infusing

Blood Administration

Giving blood correctly is one of the most important competencies. Hospitals demand nurses be 100% competent in this skill, and it is one of the skills that nursing students are not allowed to perform. One of the continuing deficiencies of senior nursing students was their inability to hang blood correctly. The only senior class that hung blood correctly was the class that administered blood products in every sophomore fundamentals scenario and in every med-surg simulation scenario. To increase successful student competency in hanging blood, blood administration was included in every simulation experience. This change produced an acceptable competency success rate. Therefore, a blood product (red blood cells [RBCs], platelets, fresh frozen plasma [FFP]) should be infused as part of every hospital day, as data shows this improves the student's ability to hang the blood product without error and correctly complete the complex paperwork. Most simulation vendors carry all types of blood products. If you order just one blood type (e.g., O neg), then all of the paperwork numbers will be the same and decrease the work of preparing the chart forms. Examples 2.3– 2.6 give examples of the blood paperwork students could use.

Example 2.3. Blood Transfusion Policy and Procedures

Purpose: To ensure a consistent approach to the prescribing, handling, and administration of blood and blood components and provide a framework and guidance for safe transfusion practice.

Procedures

1. A type & crossmatch is drawn and run by the lab when a blood transfusion is ordered.
2. The lab will assign a Blood Bank Number to the patient that matches the blood specimen drawn for the type

and cross and place a Blood Bank ID Band with this number on it on the patient.

3. Using the Consent for Transfusion of Blood or Blood Products Form, the patient's consent is obtained and witnessed. In the event that the patient is unable to sign the consent form and the transfusion is determined to be emergent, two physicians must document the need for the transfusion in the chart.
4. The nurse ensures that the patient has appropriate intravenous access to receive blood (18- or 20-gauge peripheral IV or central line access).
5. When the blood or blood product is ready for infusion, the Blood Product Issue Form/Worksheet is completed and brought to the Blood Bank. The Blood Bank will issue the blood or blood products and a Blood Transfusion Record.
6. Before the blood product is hung, two RNs must go to the bedside with the patient's blood/blood product and the Blood Transfusion Record. They will verify that the following information is consistent between the patient's Blood Bank ID Band, the Blood Transfusion Record, and the bag of Blood/Blood product:
   a. The patient's name
   b. The blood bank number
   c. The medical record number
   d. The patient's blood type
   e. The donor's blood type
   f. The donor's unit number
   g. The expiration date for the blood/blood product
7. Once the identification process is completed, both nurses will sign the Blood Transfusion Record certifying that it is the correct blood for the patient.
8. The blood product must be hung within 30 minutes of the issue time of the Blood Bank.
9. Packed cells and FFP are administered with a Y set that will enable both the blood product and an IV bag of 0.9% sodium chloride to be hung or 2 units of FFP. FFP may also be hung with one spike tubing and hung without the bag of sodium chloride. Platelets are in a 50 mL syringe and are IV pushed slowly. Flush with normal saline before and after the infusion.

10. The blood/FFP are to be administered with an infusion pump at a rate determined by the healthcare provider and the patient's condition and must be completely infused within 4 hours.
11. Vital signs are taken 15 minutes after the blood/FFP in the tubing has actually entered the patient's vein. Vital signs are monitored every 30 minutes during the infusion and 60 minutes after the infusion is complete.
12. The patient is to be monitored closely for any sign of reaction:
    a. Complaints of back pain
    b. Dark urine
    c. Chills
    d. Dizziness
    e. Fever
    f. Skin flushing
    g. Shortness of breath
    h. Itching
13. If any sign of a reaction occurs, the transfusion is to be stopped immediately, and the IV access is to be maintained. The physician is to be notified. The blood tubing and blood bag are to be sent to the lab.

Example 2.4. Consent for Transfusion of Blood or Blood Products

My physician, Dr. ____________________, has explained to me, _______________, the general nature of my condition and has informed me that a blood or blood derivative transfusion is or may be medically indicated in my case. I understand that the procedure, risks, and alternatives:

A. Description of procedure: Blood or a blood product is introduced into one of your veins, commonly in the arm, using a sterile intravenous needle. The transfusion may be whole blood, plasma, or some other blood product. The amount transfused is a judgment the physician will make.

B. Risks: Transfusion in a common procedure. Blood and its derivatives are carefully screened and subjected to rigorous testing. Basically, two levels of risks are involved:
   1. Minor and temporary reactions are not uncommon, including a slight bruise in the area where the needle pierces your skin. Non-serious reactions to the transfused material include headache, fever, itching, or rash.
   2. A serious reaction to the transfused material is possible but unlikely. Such a risk would include the danger of contracting infectious diseases. However, ALL BLOOD IS SCREENED to minimize the risk of a reaction and is specifically tested for any evidence of hepatitis or HIV/AIDS prior to transfusion. Transfusion of blood of the wrong type can be fatal, but this is highly unlikely given the fact that your blood is cross matched with the blood to be transfused prior to transfusion.

C. Alternatives: There is no effective alternative to a transfusion.
   1. Autologous donation: I understand that in some instances, it may be possible to donate one's own blood for elective medical procedures or to salvage one's own blood during some surgical procedures.
   2. Directed donation: I understand that in some cases it is possible to arrange for directed donation (donations from friends or relatives). These directed donations have not been demonstrated to be safer than blood from volunteer blood supply.

The above has been fully explained to me. I understand the factors bearing on the decision whether to authorize a transfusion of blood or blood products. I have no questions that have not been answered to my full satisfaction. I hereby consent to the receipt of such blood or blood products transfusion as my physician may decide is necessary or advisable in the course of my treatment.

____________	____________	____________
Witness	Date	Patient's Signature or Patient's Legal Representative

Example 2.5. Blood Product Issue Form

____
Date of Permit

**INFORMATION REQUIRED FOR UNIT PICKUP FROM BLOOD BANK

** Patient hospital sticker <u>or</u>:
** Pt Name ______________________________
** MR# ______________________________
**DOB ______________________________

** Blood Bank bracelet # (BB#) __________ (for PRBCs only)
** Blood Product Requested:
_______ PRBCs (Packed Red Blood Cells)
_______ Pheresis Platelets
_______ Thawed Plasma
_______ Cryoprecipitate
_______ Other ______________________________

	DATE/ TIME	B/P	TEMP	PULSE	RESP
** PRE V/S (30 minutes or less prior to start of transfusion)					
PRE MEDS (To be given at least 30 minutes prior to start of transfusion)					
UNIT# ____________ TIME ISSUED FROM BLOOD BANK ________ (Blood to be infused < 4 hours from this time)					
15 MIN V/S					
COMPLETION V/S					

CALL BLOOD BANK <u>AND</u> ORDERING PHYSICIAN IF ANY PROBLEMS

Example 2.6. Blood Transfusion Record

Name	Patient ABO/RH
BB#	Donor ABO/RH
MR#	Donor Unit #
Room	Expiration Date
Physician	Cross-Match
Date	Component
Tech	Volume
Comments	Units/Pooled
	Acc #

Issued Date/Time ______________________________

BEDSIDE VERIFICATION

Before administering this unit to ______________ MR# ________

We have verified in the patient's presence that the patient's name and hospital number are identical on the unit compatibility label, wrist band, and transfusion record, that the blood bank unit number and the blood type on transfusion record, unit compatibility label, and blood bank unit are identical, that the unit is normal in appearance and has not expired, and that the physician order has been verified by the people listed below.

Date ______________________ Transfusionist ________________

Witness ____

IN CASE OF TRANSFUSION REACTION	**TRANSFUSION REACTION SYMPTOMS**
1. Stop transfusion immediately, keep IV line open. 2. Notify Blood Bank personnel.	SHOCK CHILLS DYSPNEA NAUSEA PAIN AT INFUSION SITE FEVER (2° ABOVE BASELINE) HEADACHE ABNORMAL BLEEDING

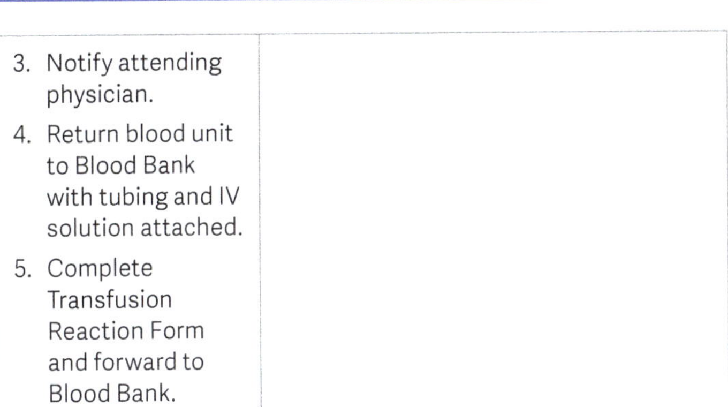

3. Notify attending physician. 4. Return blood unit to Blood Bank with tubing and IV solution attached. 5. Complete Transfusion Reaction Form and forward to Blood Bank.	

Two nurses must take the unit of blood and the Blood Bank issue form and check transfusion record with blood bag comparing patient's name, medical record number (MR#), blood bank bracelet number (BB #), ABO/RH, donor unit number, and expiration date **AT THE BEDSIDE**. Document that patient verbalized their FULL NAME and birth date. These two nurses must sign the form verifying that the blood is the correct unit for this patient.

Summary

Changing a fundamentals course and incorporating deliberate practice alone will not impact retention of learning at graduation. Deliberate practice must be inserted into all simulation experiences when new skills are taught, and mastery videos need to be incorporated for select skills. To reinforce retention of learning, all the skills taught during the fundamental course should be included in the next semester's simulation experience. This provides data on retention of learning going forward from the fundamentals course. In addition to reinforcement, continuing skills helps identify students who require remediation and skills that might require a different approach to sustain mastering. Skills can also be taught in steps. For example, if you teach intermittent urinary catheterization in a fundamentals course, the next semester's simulation could include insertion of an indwelling urinary catheter with a mastery video assignment and continue with these skills in simulations until graduation.

Employers frequently note that new graduates in nursing are weak in critical thinking and skill performance. Using simulation and deliberate practice to introduce nursing skills is one of the first steps to increase retention of learning in skill performance. Students in a simulation course fear having to perform skills in front of fellow students and faculty. Until this fear is mediated by the process of deliberate practice, students may not be ready to focus on the steps of critical thinking. This methodology increases retention of learning, which can be the first step toward critical thinking. This chapter introduced the value of deliberate practice in allowing students to perform skills repeatedly with the tools of step-by-step instructions and videos, as well as expert comments from faculty. Using simulation as an approach to teach fundamentals creates an environment that allows students to work within a realistic hospital setting and allows faculty to include many approaches to learning.

References

Clapper, T. C., & Kardong-Edgren, S. (2012). Using deliberate practice and simulation to improve nursing skills. *Clinical Simulation in Nursing, 8,* e109–e113.

Ericsson, K. A. (2008). Deliberate practice and acquisition of expert performance: A general overview. *Academic Emergency Medicine, 15,* 988–994.

Fater, K. H. (2013). Gap analysis: *A method to assess core competency development in the curriculum. Nursing Education Perspectives, 34*(2), 101–105.

INACSL Standards Committee. (2021). Healthcare Simulation Standards of Best Practice Professional Development. *Clinical Simulation in Nursing, 58,* 5–8. *https://doi.org/10.1016/j.ecns.2021.08.007*

Johnson, C. E., Kimble, L. P., Gunby, S. S., & Davis, A. H. (2020). Using deliberate practice and simulation for psychomotor skill competency acquisition and retention: A mixed-methods Study. *Nurse Educator, 45*(3), 150–154.

McIlvoy, L., & McMahan, J. (2017, June 22–24). *Incorporating student simulation outcomes into a school of nursing plan of assessment of student learning* [poster presentation]. International Nursing Association of Clinical Simulation and Learning Conference, Washington, DC, United States.

McIlvoy, L., & McMahan, J. (2020, December 1–3). *Utilizing next gen clinical judgment action model in simulation* [poster presentation]. NLN Summit, Orlando, FL, United States.

CHAPTER 3

Determination of Program, Course, and Student Needs to Be Used as Simulation Objectives

Learning Outcomes

- Clarify national nursing program accreditation.
- Determine the percentage of simulation hours within the total number of clinical hours your nursing program is permitted by your state's board of nursing.
- Appraise the NCLEX-RN Program Reports as an assessment tool.
- Explain the value of having students list their own educational needs.

To be successful, simulation must be based on what your nursing program requires. What courses would benefit from being paired with simulation? In what areas are your students the weakest? What important clinical situations are unavailable to your students locally? Which courses have the highest failure rates? Are there safety or communication issues? This chapter discusses these questions and more, the types of assessment data you need, the tools to assist in gathering it, and how simulation can help you with both program and course assessment/objectives and, ultimately, program accreditation.

Determining Program Needs

There are many requirements that nursing programs must meet to remain qualified by accreditors, their State Board of Nursing, possibly a university, local healthcare facilities, and of course the public. Below are the factions to be considered when examining the requirements for simulation programs.

Program Accreditation

Accreditation programs were established to ensure that schools of nursing have programs that are engaged in effective instructional practices. Before sitting for the National Council Licensure Examination-Registered Nurses (NCLEX-RN), candidates must have graduated from an accredited program. There are two major national accreditation bodies: the Commission on Collegiate Nursing Education (CCNE) and the Accreditation Commission for Education in Nursing (ACEN). CCNE accredits baccalaureate, graduate, and Doctor of Nursing Practice programs, whereas ACEN accredits all types of nursing programs. PhD programs are accredited by specialty, national, or regional accreditation bodies.

Both CCNE and ACEN have standards and defining essentials or criterion to determine if a school meets the benchmarks established for quality in nursing education. While ACEN's (2020) Curriculum Standard requires that end-of-program student learning outcomes (senior level) are completed for accreditation, CCNE's (2018) Curriculum Standard requires student learning outcomes achievement with no stipulation as to end of program. It is interesting that the term "simulation" is rarely mentioned in either manual. Accreditation organizations agree that assessment data used to guide program decision making is at the center of accreditation. Simulation data, especially end-of-program simulation data, can provide evidence of program effectiveness as well as drive program improvement. However, the ultimate evidence of program effectiveness remains the NCLEX-RN pass rate.

National Council of State Boards of Nursing (NCSBN)

The NCSBN is responsible for creating and administering the NCLEX-RN. Pass rates on the NCLEX-RN must be greater than 80% to prove that nursing programs are effective and therefore worthy of national accreditation (ACEN, 2020; CCNE, 2018). As of April 2023, the NCLEX-RN Test Plan will incorporate clinical judgment into the Client Needs categories (NCSBN, 2023b). This inclusion is based on the development of the framework of the NCSBN's Next Gen Clinical Judgment Measurement Model (CJMM; see Chapter 1 for more information on the model). There are a multitude of teaching modalities available to help prepare students for this addition to the Test Plan. Simulation offers a modality that brings all six of the CJMM measurable clinical decision-making steps into focus. To make decisions on simulation program objectives, course and student assessments should be completed.

State Boards of Nursing Simulation Rules

In 2014, the NCSBN performed a national study on the effectiveness of simulation when compared to clinical experience. Their results indicated that 50% of clinical experiences could be replaced with simulation experiences without a change in the outcomes of knowledge, competency, and critical thinking when students were followed up to 6 months postgraduation (Hayden et al., 2014). Since the publication of this article, each state's board of nursing has the autonomy to set the percentage of clinical hours that may be substituted with simulation hours for their state. The 2022 Educational Survey of 50 states and 7 U.S. territories by the NCSBN (2023a) answered the following question: "What is the maximum amount of clinical hours that may be replaced by simulation hours?" (p. 47). The following was determined: 19% do not address simulation hours, 4% allow unlimited amount, 1% allow up to 75%, 61% allow up to 50%, 2% allow up to 30%, and 12% allow up to 25%. Since the publication of the hallmark article, the NCSBN (Alexander et al., 2015) have developed Simulation Guidelines for Prelicensure Nursing Programs. These guidelines contain preparatory checklists for both the simulation program and the faculty, which are included below.

NCSBN Program Preparation Checklist

- The school has created a framework that provides adequate resources (fiscal, human, and material) to support the simulation.
- Policies and procedures are in place to ensure quality-consistent simulation experiences for the students.
- The simulation program has an adequate number of dedicated trained simulation faculty members to support the learners in simulation-based experiences.
- The program has job descriptions for simulation faculty members/facilitators.
- The program has a plan for orienting simulation faculty members to their roles.
- The program uses a needs assessment to determine what scenarios to use.
- The simulation program provides subject-matter expertise for each scenario debriefing.
- The program and faculty members incorporate the INACSL Standards of Best Practice: Simulation.
- The program has appropriate designated physical space for education, storage, and debriefing.
- The faculty members have a process for identifying what equipment or relevant technologies are needed for meeting program objectives.
- The program has adequate equipment and supplies to create a realistic patient care environment.
- The faculty use evaluative feedback for quality improvement of the simulation program.
- The administration has a long-range plan for anticipated use of simulation in the forthcoming years.

Source: NCSBN Program Preparation Checklist." Copyright © 2016 by National Council of State Boards of Nursing, Inc. Reprinted with permission.

NCSBN Faculty Preparation Checklist

- The simulation program is based on educational theories associated with simulation, such as experiential learning theory.
- The faculty members are prepared by following the INACSL Standards of Best Practice: Simulation.
- A tool for evaluating simulation-based learning experiences has been designed based on the INASCL Standards of Best Practice: Simulation evaluation methods.
- The program curriculum sets clear objectives and expected outcomes for each simulation-based experience, which are communicated to students prior to each simulation activity.
- The faculty members are prepared to create a learning environment that encourages active learning, repetitive practice, and reflection and to provide appropriate support throughout each activity.
- The faculty members are prepared to use facilitation methods congruent with simulation objectives/expected outcomes.
- The program utilizes a standardized method of debriefing observed simulation using a Socratic methodology.
- A rubric has been developed to evaluate the students' acquisition of KSAs (knowledge, skills, and attitudes) throughout the program.
- The program has established a method of sharing student performance with clinical faculty.
- The program collects and retains evaluation data regarding the effectiveness of the facilitator.
- The program collects and retains evaluation data regarding the effectiveness of the simulation experience.
- The program provides a means for faculty members to participate in simulation-related professional development, such as webinars, conferences, journals, clubs, readings,

and certifications such as certified health care simulation educator (CHSE), and participation in NLN Sim Leaders/ Sigma Theta Tau International (STTI) Nurse Faculty Leadership Academy (NFLA) with a focus on simulation.

Source: NCSBN Faculty Preparation Checklist." Copyright © 2016 by National Council of State Boards of Nursing, Inc. Reprinted with permission.

NCLEX-RN Reports

Another avenue of data that could point to program needs are the NCLEX-RN reports from the NCSBN. For a fee, you can order these based on when your graduates sit for the exam (https://www.ncsbn.org/exams/exam-statistics-and-publications/nclex-program-reports.page). If you graduate students more than once a year, reports can be ordered covering more than one time frame. These reports give the results for your program on the NCLEX-RN Test Plan: 5 phases of the Nursing Process, 8 categories of Human Functioning, 10 categories of Health Alterations, 6 stages of maturity, and the 4 aspects of Stress, Adaptation, and Coping. The report gives you comparison data for your jurisdiction, all programs like yours, and the national data. Additionally, it lists your last year's results for comparison. The most important data for comparison would be the national data, as programs should strive to be above the national average. The data is not given in percentages but rather in percentile ranks based on graduates' performance. Purchasing this report annually will provide your program with longitudinal data that can highlight problems and successes and allow for an improvement plan for a specific problem in a client need. A specific area that needs improvement would benefit from combined didactic and simulation approaches.

Program Objectives

Patient Safety: Medication Administration

Patient safety is a major concern that appears in multiple national organization's statements and guidelines, such as the National Institutes of Health, Centers for Disease Control and Prevention, and Agency for Healthcare Research and Quality, to name a few. Patient safety objectives should be threaded throughout the nursing program. Every simulation should have the same approach for medication errors. Students should fill out an incident report, and a plan for improvement should be developed for the student(s). Sometime errors are a combination of factors that contribute to the error. These medication errors should be examined, as they are an important flag that something is missing. The effectiveness of the improvement plan for these students is a necessary step to ensure both student and program success. Below are examples of the policy on medication incidents and medication errors.

Clinical Simulation Medication Incident Policy

Purpose: To ensure that students are competent and safe in administering medications in clinical simulation.

Policy: Students who make an error during medication administration will be required to fill out a Medication Incident Report.

1. The student will:
    a. Attach patient label in the appropriate box.
    b. Fill in date.
    c. List the name of all of the students involved in the medication administration error.
    d. List the patient's name.
    e. Place a check on the line of the type of medication error.
    f. Place a check on the line if any of the other medication incidents occurred.
    g. Write a statement about how the incident/error could have been prevented.
    h. Write a statement explaining how the incident/error was corrected.
    i. Write a statement stating the impact of the incident/error on the patient.
2. Faculty will complete the action that was taken as a result of the incident/error.
    a. If incident/error was caused by a failure of one of the five rights of medication administration, the

student(s) will be placed on a clinical contract and their clinical faculty will be notified.

   b. If the incident/error is the first occurrence and recognized by the student before the end of the simulation and the appropriate medical provider is notified, the student must still fill out the Medication Incident Report but will not be placed on a clinical contract.
   c. A second incident/error occurring during medication administration either in clinical simulation or in clinical agency (or documentation of a prior medication incident/error) may result in an unsatisfactory grade in the practicum.
3. Both faculty and student will sign the report, and it will be placed in the student's file in the Nursing Office.

Clinical Simulation Medication Incident Report

Date: ______ **Student(s) Involved:** ____________________

____

Patient Name: ______________________________

Type of Medication Error:	Other Medication Incident:
Wrong Medication	___ Medication not given
___ Wrong Dosage	___ Medication inadvertently rendered unusable
___ Wrong Patient	___ Newly prescribed medication not initiated
___ Wrong Route	___ Medication not available
___ Wrong Time	___ Medication refused

How could this incident or error have been prevented?

____

____

How was this incident or error corrected?

____

____

How was the patient impacted by this incident or error?

____

____

Performance improvement plan initiated by faculty:

____

____

____

Faculty Signature ____________ **Student Signature** ____________

Patient Safety: Patient Identification/Communication

The first step in any interaction with a patient is to determine that the identification of the individual is correct in terms of whatever medication, treatment, and so on has been ordered for a specific patient. This is done by requesting identification verification from the patient by two methods, most commonly name and birth date as requested by the Joint Commission and verifying information against the patient's ID bracelet. For patients who are unable to verbalize information, the ID bracelet on the patient is checked for name and birth date against the chart or Electronic Medical Record. Compliance for this safety communication needs verification, and compliance data can be produced via clinical simulation.

Patient Safety: Patient Communication

Communication is another objective that requires program-level consideration. Nursing communication skills with healthcare providers (HCPs) can adversely impact patient safety if communication is lacking important information or delivered either too aggressively or passively. Most nursing programs introduce the ISBAR (Identify, Situation, Background, Assessment, and Recommendation) framework as a tool to guide communication. However, to achieve mastery of this technique requires considerable practice in many nursing specialties. Students are rarely allowed to communicate with HCPs during clinical, as they are unlicensed personnel.

Both patient safety and communication objectives can be inserted into any simulation scenario, despite level of student. This ongoing practice over years in a reality-based simulated healthcare environment allows time for students to acquire mastery and provides the data that confirms it. These communication skills are examples of data that should be followed by a program assessment committee.

Determining Course Needs

Almost any clinical situation can be experienced in a simulated environment. Currently, many nursing programs are using obstetrical simulations, as they cannot place all their students in an appropriate clinical area. If one of your primary program outcomes is focused on diversity, this could be built into simulation scenarios to both educate students and provide valuable data on student knowledge and behaviors.

Courses with matching didactic and clinical content would be appropriate choices for clinical simulation. The simulation can share the clinical objectives or have objectives that are more specific under the clinical objectives. Courses that have high failure rates should be considered for simulation. This would provide an avenue where the content of the course could be provided with a different methodology that provides an active environment, especially if the scenarios involve small groups of students. This teaches teamwork and lessens anxiety while exposing students to the course's educational priorities.

Faculty should determine which kind of simulation would be beneficial, such as an interprofessional approach involving more than one class, other campus programs, and even community participants. This would create connections within the faculty and between departments and/or communities that would benefit everyone. Mass casualty simulations are an example of this type of situation.

Data from the NCLEX-RN report would help identify content from specific courses that students struggled with as a group in their examination. This content could be addressed in a variety of ways within simulation. Again, courses that do not offer the best clinical sites could benefit from a simulation that would specifically address the information and reaction to problems that the course presents.

Determining Student Needs

What areas of knowledge are perceived as missing or weak by students in terms of course content and psychomotor skills at the end of each semester or year? Students will tell you what skills they are weak in performing; however, after faculty assessment, skills that students think they have mastered may demonstrate a lack of knowledge and technique. Without comfortably performing skills, students become anxious and cannot focus on the objective of the scenario. Even in situations where students master required psychomotor skills before they move forward in the curriculum, there will be students who fulfilled the criteria for mastering but lack retention the following semester. Having a method to acquire retention of learning is helpful in understanding student needs. To reinforce mastery of psychomotor skills, it is helpful to have a methodology that promotes such mastery. The theory of deliberate practice was introduced in Chapter 2. Creating a standard methodology in nursing clinical and simulation programs will facilitate student mastery of psychomotor skills throughout the program. Designing simulation experiences that reinforce learning will aid in knowledge retention.

Summary

It is advantageous to assess program, course, and student needs to develop clinical simulation objectives. Program outcomes are commonly based on the mission and goals of the parent institution, faculty outcomes, and the national standards, guidelines, and competencies that are applicable to undergraduate nursing programs. The two national agendas of patient safety and communication require specific education that is easily inserted into all simulations to reinforce learning and provide appropriate longitudinal data as students progress through the program. Course-level needs are easily converted into simulation objectives, as both are centered on student learning. Students' knowledge and skills needs may require a remediation plan. How to use assessment data in developing specific simulation objectives as part of the simulation scenario design will be covered in the next chapter.

References

Accreditation Commission for Education in Nursing. (2020). *ACEN accreditation manual*. https://www.acenursing.org/accreditation-manual-july-2020/

Alexander, M., Durham, C., Hooper, J., Jeffries, P., Goldman, N., Kardong-Edgren, S. Kesten, K. S., Spector, N., Tagliareni, E., Radtke, B., & Tillman, C. (2015). NCSBN simulation guidelines for prelicensure nursing programs. *Journal of Nursing Regulation*, *6*(3), 39–42.

Commission on Collegiate Nursing Education. (2018). *CCNE accreditation, standards, procedures, & guidelines*. American Association of Colleges of Nursing. https://www.aacnnursing.org/ccne-accreditation/accreditation-resources/standards-procedures-guidelines

Hayden, J. K., Smiley, R. A., Alexander, M., Kardong-Edgren, S., & Jeffries, P. R. (2014). The NCSBN National Simulation Study: A longitudinal, randomized, controlled study replacing clinical hours with simulation in prelicensure nursing education. *Journal of Nursing Regulation*, *5*(Suppl. 2), S3–S64.

National Council of State Boards of Nursing. (2016a). *NCSBN simulation faculty preparation checklist*. https://www.ncsbn.org/public-files/16_Simulation_Faculty_Checklist.pdf

National Council of State Boards of Nursing. (2016b). *NCSBN simulation program preparation checklist*. https://www.ncsbn.org/public-files/16_Simulation_Program_Checklist.pdf

National Council of State Boards of Nursing. (2023a). *2022 Education Survey*. https://www.ncsbn.org/public-files/Education_Survey_2022.pdf

National Council of State Boards of Nursing (2023b). *Next Generation NCLEX-RN Test Plan*. https://www.nclex.com/files/2023_RN_Test%20Plan_English_FINAL.pdf

CHAPTER 4

Clinical Simulation Scenario Design That Incorporates CJMM

Learning Outcomes

- Describe the appropriate process for creating a learning objective.
- Explain how to remodel simulation scenarios to include the CJMM.
- Differentiate between the types of scenarios used with different levels of students.
- Apply the information presented to build a scenario design template.
- Develop a scenario using CJMM.

The first step in designing a simulation scenario is the determination of the specific program, course, and student objectives you wish the scenario to address and which participants are appropriate. As covered in the previous chapter, the program objectives (e.g., safety and communication) are embedded in all scenarios. Course objectives are specific to each course and faculty, may be paired with didactic objectives, and include student psychomotor skills when applicable.

Student objectives are frequently tied to the retention of learning. The scenario specifics are driven by the objectives, faculty numbers, equipment availability, the type of ideal patient (standard or mannequin), the appropriate fidelity, and the setting (within lab/simulation room, classroom, or community).

Objectives and Expected Outcomes

Once the needs assessment is completed, objectives are developed that aim to achieve the outcome that addresses the appropriate need. Program outcomes are relevant to accreditation, national goals of patient safety, standards, guidelines, and competencies. Course outcomes are tied to student attainment of specific knowledge and skills. Student outcomes are centered on retention of learning (INACSL Standards Committee, 2021b). Objectives should be clear, meaningful, and attainable. Using the acronym "SMART" reminds writers to create objectives that are specific, measurable, achievable, relevant, and timely) (INACSL Standards Committee, 2021b). An objective should also be stated using Bloom's taxonomy, which was developed by Bloom in 1956. In 2001 the taxonomy was revised to a taxonomy of teaching, learning, and assessment (Anderson & Krathwohl, 2001). This taxonomy contains six categories that increase in complexity: remember, understand, apply, analyze, evaluate, and create. Under each category, there is a list of "action verbs" that indicate the level of thinking presented by the objective (https://bloomstaxonomy.net/). For example, a student learning objective for a fundamental course simulation lab where they learn how to prime IV tubing might be "At the end of this course the student will be able to: Demonstrate in a master video how to insert IV tubing into an IV bag of fluids and prime the tubing with IV fluid following the School of Nursing's step-by-step directions without error." The verb of "demonstrate" falls under the category of *apply*, which is defined as the ability to "carry out or use a procedure in a given situation" (Anderson & Krathwohl, 2001, p. 97).

Clinical Simulation Scenario Design

Simulation scenario design is complex. After the outcome and participants are selected, which level of fidelity will facilitate the achievement of the objectives is determined. A content expert is needed to ensure that the scenario is developed with the appropriate knowledge content and level for the chosen participants. The scenario designs discussed here use a mannequin in the role of the patient. It is important that the six actions of the CJMM be incorporated and linked to outcomes in these simulation scenarios.

One of the most common issues in hospitals is the inability of new graduate nurses to function at the level that allows them to recognize when patients are experiencing a negative event and intervene (i.e., failure to rescue). The CJMM describes the steps of how nurses can be taught clinical judgment. The brain stores memories of learning that occurs during clinical simulations that are realistic and focused on clinical judgment. When nurses are faced with real-life clinical situations that requires clinical judgment, they are more likely to access the knowledge that was gained in a similar situation, such as a simulation experience that involved clinical judgment (Morris et al, 1977).

There are two levels of scenarios, one at the junior level and one at the senior level. The junior-level scenario is suitable for students undergoing their first experiences in acute care, and the senior-level scenario is appropriate for end-of-program assessment. Chapter 2 discussed the simulation of fundamentals and psychomotor skills that are applicable to first-year students.

The complexity of simulation scenarios are such that they are frequently compared to producing a Broadway play. Most faculty use a template to keep track of all aspects of the scenario design and ensure that all the parts are included in the planning. There are multiple examples of scenario templates on the internet and in books on simulation; however, none were found that use the CJMM for their development. Examples of scenario templates for senior- and junior-level nursing students that emphasize Bloom's taxonomy in the objectives are provided below. They are based on courses that include clinical experiences and use simulation as part of those clinical hours.

Building Junior- and Senior-Level Scenarios and Using Templates to Produce the Scenario Map

The junior-level type of scenario involves the care of two patients in the same room by teams of two students for each patient. Each patient requires the psychomotor skills that were taught the previous semester in fundamentals to assess retention of learning. These patients are medical/surgical patients with a variety of diagnoses that are covered during the didactic class. The problem that is introduced is either a safety issue (patient ordered a medication with an existing allergy), an abnormal lab (requiring a blood product), an abnormal temperature or BP, or another issue that requires communication with a healthcare professional (HCP) using ISBAR (identify, situation, background, assessment, recommendation).

The senior-level type of scenario incorporates the CJMM in their development and involves recognizing the signs and symptoms of a given diagnosis and being able to differentiate between what the patient's condition was and what has changed and the corresponding implications. These scenarios also last up to an hour and work best with a team of 2–4 students caring for the patient in a critical care environment. Each student draws a card for their randomly assigned role. Routinely, these roles are documenter/communicator, IV management, lab draw/glucose management/dressing change, and PEG medication/feeding management. These scenarios involve the performance of complex psychomotor skills, documentation of care, and communication with an HCP using the ISBAR method. After the start of the scenario, the mannequin only responds to an action (or lack of needed action) by the students. Adequate time is given to allow students to think, discuss as a team, and determine action.

Part 1 of the Clinical Simulation Scenario Template establishes the outcome and objectives based on the CJMM. The participants are described, the fidelity is established, and a content expert is identified. The patient's health data is described, supplying a past and current medical history. Moulage and equipment that is required are listed. The program objectives of safety and communication are included in all scenarios. The specific course scenarios are determined by faculty and in line with the didactic course objectives. Two to three objectives specific to the scenario are appropriate. The fidelity of the mannequin is determined by finances and the ability to simulates reality. For senior-level critical care, ideally, a high-fidelity mannequin would be used. However, these scenarios can be run with a skills mannequin and a lot of "magic" (see Chapter 7).

The senior-level template—Clinical Simulation Scenario Template (Part 2)—generally uses an admission (ADM) scenario as students inconsistently get to participate in this high-stress complex phase of care during clinical experiences. The orders are listed on the template and include all the requirements for new admissions: diagnosis, labs, consents needed, medications, IV fluids and rates, dressing changes, diet, mobility, oxygen, and so on. The medications from the orders are placed on the Medication Administration Record (MAR).

Documentation can involve either Electronic Health Records (EHRs) or paper charts. Arguments can be made for either. There is a shift toward not allowing students to chart in hospital EHRs for a variety of reasons. However, purchasing a product from nursing education vendors can be financially unrealistic and can be complex when it comes to entering orders and other duties. Yet if hospitals won't let students access their EHRs, purchasing one may be the only way to provide this invaluable skill. On the other hand, having students that have not been exposed to a paper chart can handicap them when hospital EHRs are not working and a paper chart is substituted.

The scenario template lists the diagnosis, the student learning outcomes of the CJMM with Bloom's taxonomy of learning levels, participants, level of fidelity, and the content expert. It also lists the program-level student performance behaviors (SPBs) that should have been exhibited during the scenario.

Clinical Simulation Scenario Template (Part 1)

Course: ______________ **Patient Name:** ________________

Simulation Scenario Student Learning Outcomes:

Students will successfully care for a patient diagnosed with ______________________ experiencing negative physiological events by:

- Recognizing and analyzing cues (Remember/Analyze Levels)
- Generating a hypothesis of the pathophysiological event (Create Level)

- Performing the action of notifying a health care provider (Apply Level)
- Taking action correctly when carrying out orders (Apply Level)
- Evaluating the outcome (Evaluate level)

Participants:

Level of Fidelity and Choice of Mannequin:

Content Expert:

At the end of the scenario, students will have demonstrated the following PROGRAM OBJECTIVES OF SAFETY AND COMMUNICATION SKILLS:

- Appropriate identification of patient
- Appropriate safety and communication skills
- Precise medication administration
- Appropriate assessment skills
- Correct performance of specific psychomotor skills
- Organizes for and implements discussion with HCP
- Determination of outcome

Specific Course Scenario Objectives

1. ______________________________________
2. ______________________________________

   ____

A worksheet of information is also created for required paperwork/ ID bands/MARs and any supplies needed in the room as well as wounds, tubes, and IV sites that would be required. The fidelity of these mannequins can be low to moderate. Skills trainers are the easiest. To have monitors and patients speaking, see Chapter 7.

Part 2 of the scenario template is where the actual scenario progression is written. The information at the top is helpful in setting up the patient for the scenario. The Scenario Progression Template has two columns: Student Performance Behaviors (SPBs) and Mannequin Response. First, under SPBs, the program safety objectives are listed for all scenarios that have students verify that all of the listed are correct. Nursing practice for registered nurses is driven by healthcare provider (HCP) orders, and students require an understanding of this caveat. Sources like the media often show "nurses" independently performing interventions that normally require HCP orders. Of course, the opposite is also true, as nurses are given orders by physicians for interventions within nursing autonomy. Students are introduced to the concept of HCP orders early in nursing school, but it is during early simulation that conceptualization occurs (see Chapter 2 for techniques to introduce orders during early simulation). This is why scenarios start with checking orders and "signing them off," which is a legal act of accepting responsibility that each order has been completed. Documentation is accomplished through flow sheets with paper charts or EHRs to introduce students to charting while caring for a patient.

Students must identify themselves. The rest of the columns are listed as student-expected performance behaviors. These behaviors are categorized under the "CJMM" and "Safety." Recognizing a cue that something is not as it should be is the first step. Cues are given for the problem from a variety of sources (e.g., vital signs, focused assessment, lab values, patient statements, etc.). Once students have analyzed the nature of the problem based on the cues, they form hypotheses of what is happening, prioritize the hypotheses, and take action by notifying the HCP. They use ISBAR to notify the HCP of the cues, state their hypothesis, and recommend actions. After completing the ordered actions, they evaluate the outcome.

Part 2 lists the specifics that are included in all scenarios. At the top of the form, all of the setup information for the day of simulation is listed, making it easier and faster. You can add information such as breathing tubes, oxygen/ventilator settings, lab values, arterial lines, and so on. The specific course scenario objectives are listed here. For example, a patient diagnosed with exacerbation of heart failure might have the student learning objective of "Recognizes the signs and symptoms of worsening heart failure and determines, discusses, and implements a plan of treatment with the HCP."

See below for an example of an actual senior-level scenario progression. The first form is the blank template and the second is an example of an actual patient scenario. A student's ability to use the steps of critical thinking can be determined in these scenarios as well as provide a vital measurement of retention of learning.

Clinical Simulation Scenario Template (PART 2)

Patient Name: ____________ **Age:** ________ **WT:** ________

Dx: ________________________________

IV Sites/Type & Tubes: ________________________________

IV Fluids & Rate: ________________________________

Drips: ________________________________

Blood: ________________________________

Dressings: ________________________________

Scenario Progression Template

Student Required Actions: Student performance behaviors	**Response** Driven by faculty per scenario AND in response to student action
-Verifies (Evaluation Level) **SAFETY: Retention of Learning Measurement** • MD Orders • Patient ID bracelet against chart • Patient name and DOB • IV pumps working and correct fluids hanging • Side rails are up • HOB elevated if appropriate **-Introduces themselves**	**Beginning vital signs on monitor:** Heart rhythm ________ HR ____ BP ______ RR ______ SaO2 ______ ABP ______ PAP ______ Temp: Peripheral __________ Breath Sounds __________
-Performs physical assessment **-Assesses pain (verbal and nonverbal)** **CHS, SAFETY: Retention of Learning Measurement** **-Performs ordered nursing care** **SAFETY: Retention of Learning Measurement** • Dressing changes	**Self-generated recognition of <u>Cue, Hypothesis, & Solution</u> (CHS) where a previous order covers the treatment such as pain complaint: pain medicine given then reevaluated, abnormal blood sugar: treated with sliding scale.**

• Tube care and feedings
• Scheduled medication administration
• PRN medication administration
• If applicable
  ○ Blood sugar checks
  ○ Scheduled lab draw
  ○ Blood product administration	

-Recognizes and analyzes cues	**-Provide initial cues (such as): Labs results, changes in vital signs or assessment findings, statements from patient, medical/surgical history**

-Prioritizes hypothesis & generates solutions
• Takes action and places call to HCP using ISBAR
  ○ Identifies self and patient
  ○ Gives current problem: Vital signs, labs, assessment data, etc.
  ○ Offers recommendation
  ○ Repeats orders
	HCP: Script of questions asked and orders given

-Takes action and completes orders • Prioritizes orders • Gives medications correctly • Administers blood products following step-by-step instructions from hospital policy and procedure • Orders and performs collection of laboratory specimens • Reassesses patient condition frequently • Documents interventions appropriately	**Ends scenario**

Scenario

Patient Name: Lucy Belmont **Age:** 60 **WT:** 87 KG

Dx: Hypertension, Type II Diabetes, Colon CA

Lines & Tubes: Left Triple Lumen, Arterial line, PEG

IV Fluids: NS at 75 mL/hr **Drips:** Nitroglycerin hanging at 6 mg/min

Allergies: Codeine, Sulfa

Needed for Scenario: Nitroglycerin drip 100 MG/250 NS with tubing, Heparin drip 25,000 units/ 250 mL NS, K (potassium) 10 meq in 50 mL NS, in Nasal Cannula on at 2 Liters, AM Lab results, Right groin wound with SMALL amt blood

DOB 06-17-1960

Scenario Progression

Student Actions **Student Performance Behaviors**	**Mannequin Response** **Faculty (Health Care Provider) Communication**
-Checks MD Orders -Verifies IV pumps working and correct fluids hanging -HOB elevated 30 degrees -Puts side rails up -Introduces themselves -Checks patient name and birthdate -Hangs heparin drip -Draws BMP labs and sends to lab	**Opening Vital Signs on Monitor:** **Heart rhythm: NSR HR: 70** **ABP: 128/70 RR: 28 SaO2: 95%** **Temp: Periph 99.8** **Breath Sounds: Lots of Crackles** **Call Room: Ask if Lucy is back from Cath Lab.** • Start Heparin Protocol for Acute Coronary Syndrome will send orders and Heparin bag and her coagulation results • Draw a stat Basic Metabolic Panel and send it, please
Asks Questions	"Lucy Belmont, 6-17-60"
-Assesses Pain → -Perform physical assessment -Gives PEG meds and SQ meds -Dressing Change Gives All Meds	"I'm fine" **BP 102/48 Atrial Fib 90** **RR30 Sat 93%**

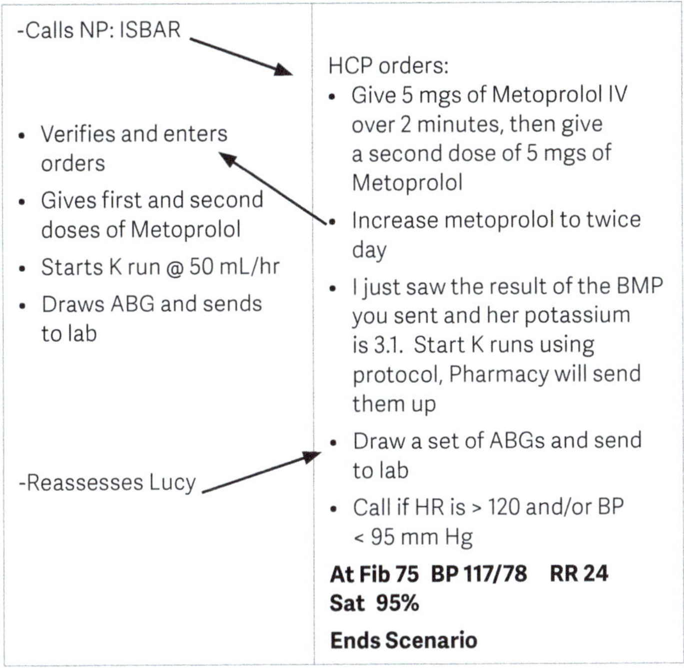

-Calls NP: ISBAR • Verifies and enters orders • Gives first and second doses of Metoprolol • Starts K run @ 50 mL/hr • Draws ABG and sends to lab -Reassesses Lucy	HCP orders: • Give 5 mgs of Metoprolol IV over 2 minutes, then give a second dose of 5 mgs of Metoprolol • Increase metoprolol to twice day • I just saw the result of the BMP you sent and her potassium is 3.1. Start K runs using protocol, Pharmacy will send them up • Draw a set of ABGs and send to lab • Call if HR is > 120 and/or BP < 95 mm Hg **At Fib 75 BP 117/78 RR 24 Sat 95%** **Ends Scenario**

Abbreviations:

HTN: Hypertension
CA: Cancer
Art: Arterial
NS: Normal Saline
NTG: Nitroglycerin
NC: Nasal Cannula
BMP: Basic Metabolic Panel
ISBAR: Identify Situation Background Assessment Recommendation
K run 10 meq Potassium in 50 mL IVPB to infuse over 1 hour
ABG: Arterial Blood Gas

Prebriefing for Juniors and Seniors

First, a confidentiality statement should be signed by all students. At the beginning of the semester, an introduction to clinical simulation is held in the junior med-surg class and senior critical care class. Slides are used to explain the type of patient and the preparation students will need to participate in, and the new psychomotor skill for that semester is demonstrated. At the end of the class on how clinical simulation runs, students return to the lab to practice the new skill. The patient's diagnosis, descriptive data, and MAR, as well as the reading assignment, are shared with students usually 3–5 days before the simulation. This gives them plenty of time to prepare. Juniors understand that all of their sophomore-level psychomotor skills will be used and they should review the master videos they made for each skill. Seniors are informed that they will have the skills of IV management using a central triple lumen catheter, IV and PEG medications, drawing from an arterial line, changing ventilator settings or oxygen modes, and sterile dressing changes in all simulations and are reminded of their week of simulation.

On the morning of the simulation, students are taken to the simulation room and review how all of the equipment works (IV pumps, feeding pumps, PCA pumps, and chest tubes). The wall mounted vital sign monitors are explained. The flow of the scenario is discussed as well as the roles. Communication among them is discussed, as everyone in the room needs to know what's going on. How to prepare for an ISBAR phone call is also reviewed. The group is told that they can call anyone for questions or help at any time just like in the hospital. The phone numbers for Pharmacy, Central Supply, and HCP are next to the phone. The clinical group (of eight) is split in half, as there are two scenarios.

Before the scenario begins, a report is given by the night nurse (faculty) The report is very complete, giving the history and diagnosis and what occurred before they arrived to the unit the orders. The patient's medical orders are reviewed as well as which labs are done, which are pending, how to use the phone, the supplies in the room, and so forth. Family and their availability are discussed. Students are encouraged to take notes. Faculty answer any questions and then leave.

Observing Simulation

The observing group of four can observe using a variety of options. They can sit in the control room and watch through the two-way mirror with faculty. Sometimes this is the only way to manage an observation experience, but faculty have to remain professional and talk with students about what is going on, why, and what they would do. With a system that telecasts the simulation to a conference room, students can watch from there and complete an observation assignment. They answer questions about things like what is going on when a vital sign changes, what action would they do, the best thing the group did, the things they would have done differently, what the most important things the group did were..., and so on.

Midsimulation Assistance to Students

Should students become "stuck" on a skill or understanding an order, the "charge nurse" makes rounds to help them problem-solve their issues. Nothing is learned when students are stressed because they can't get an IV pump to stop beeping or they can't find an "amp" of something. The charge nurse calms the students down and helps them problem-solve and continue the scenario.

Debriefing

There are multiple evidence-based techniques for debriefing available to use. The INACSL standard on the debriefing process covers the four criteria that are necessary to meet this standard of best practice (INACSL Standards Committee, 2021a): The debriefing process (1) is planned and incorporated into the simulation-based experience; (2) is constructed, designed, and/or facilitated by a person(s) or system capable and competent; (3) should encourage reflection, exploration of knowledge, and identification of performance deficits while maintaining psychological safety and confidentiality; and (4) should allow for flexibility based on different learners, identified objectives and outcomes, timeframe, and the simulation setting and be designed to promote critical thinking and reflection. A wide variety of evidence-based debriefing techniques can be found in the Reference entries for this standard.

If recording or telecasting live scenarios isn't feasible, you can debrief at the bedside using the U.S. Army's After-Action Review for Simulation Debriefing (Sawyer & Deering, 2013). This is also helpful if there is a problem, for example, with how IVPB or IV drips were hung. Allowing students to see at the bedside what they did wrong and work toward correcting it is extremely helpful.

There are seven sequential steps that include how the debriefing will occur and what it was designed to teach students. Start at the beginning of the scenario and walk through it with the students; it's easier to recall what actually occurred remembering student steps in the order they occurred. Have students discuss what evidence (cues) were used to guide hypotheses and potential interventions. Were they prepared to take action by calling the HCP, and did they use ISBAR? What was supposed to happen versus what actually happened, and why? What went well, what didn't go well, and what you would do next time are a nice wrap-up. Remember to allow them to discuss how they felt during the good and the not-so-good. It's helpful to do this at the bedside because without a video it is difficult to remember what you actually did in an hour-long simulation unless you are surrounded by the tools you used with the patient.

If you have videos that are available immediately, you can walk through the same debriefing in a separate room. Or you can combine both methods, at the bedside and using videos. The videos that are prepared by the newer sophisticated systems allow you to flag certain actions during the scenario that are helpful in focusing students on the steps of clinical judgment.

Summary

Incorporating the CJMM steps into complex and long simulation scenarios provides students with the opportunity to demonstrate their ability to deal with a patient problem during a hospital shift. For junior-level scenarios, focus is on the performance of psychomotor skills and identifying a cue and hypothesizing a simple problem (e.g., lab result, change in a vital sign, etc.). A critical care setting was used with senior-level students with scenarios redesigned to be longer and include a patient problem to be solved using the steps of the CJMM. The SPBs are the focus of each scenario. A more in-depth look at SPBs and data that demonstrates the important outcomes of this scenario design will be provided in the next chapter.

References

Anderson, L. W., & Krathwohl, D. R. (2001). *A taxonomy for learning, teaching, and assessing*. Pearson Education.

INACSL Standards Committee. (2021a, September). Healthcare Simulation Standards of Best Practice: The debriefing process. *Clinical Simulation in Nursing, 58*, 27–32. https://doi.org/10.1016/j.ecns.2021.08.011

INACSL Standards Committee. (2021b, September). Healthcare Simulation Standards of Best Practice: Outcomes and objectives. *Clinical Simulation in Nursing, 58*, 40–44. https://doi.org/10.1016/j.ecns.2021.08.013

Morris, D., Bransford, J. D., & Franks, J. J. (1977). Levels of processing versus transfer appropriate processing. *Journal of Verbal Learning and Verbal Behavior, 16*(5), 519–533.

Sawyer, T. L., & Deering, S. (2013). Adaptation of the U.S. Army's after-action review for simulation debriefing in healthcare. *Simulation in Healthcare, 8*(6), 388–397. https://doi.org/10.1097/SIH.0b013e31829ac85c

CHAPTER 5

Student Performance Behaviors as a Measure of Safety/Communication Abilities, Psychomotor Skills Retention, and Clinical Judgment

Learning Outcomes

- Determine the specific competencies of a clinical simulation scenario.
- Integrate CJMM into clinical simulation scenarios.
- Develop specific student performance behaviors (SPBs) for students in clinical simulation scenarios.
- Explain how outcomes of SPBs can be used for student, course, and program evaluation.

Nurses are required to excel in performing the psychomotor skills taught to all nursing students in a nursing fundamentals course. There is now a directive that nursing students develop clinical judgment to facilitate prioritization and develop the ability to rescue patients. The requirement for both categories is that they are evidence-based and can be measured by SPBs. The evaluation of these SPBs can be used as the method for student, course, and program assessment. This chapter discusses the development of SPBs using psychomotor skills and the layers of the NCSBN's Clinical Judgment Measurement Model (CJMM). The data that demonstrates the effectiveness of SPBs in evaluating the success of each student and simulation scenario is discussed. Examples of how to use end-of-program senior-level SPB data in formal program assessment are provided.

Evaluation of Clinical Simulation

Two important issues in nursing education are how to evaluate clinical performance and how to quantify learning from clinical simulation. The National Institutes of Health Office of Human Resources (n.d.) defines *competencies* as "the knowledge, skills, abilities, and behaviors that contribute to individual and organizational performance" (para. 1). Employing specific competencies in a clinical simulation program helps to identify the specific behaviors that you want students to demonstrate. The competencies that are applicable to the simulation discussed so far are safety, communication, retention of learning, and the six clinical judgments of the CJMM: recognizing cues, analyzing cues, prioritizing hypotheses, generating solutions, taking action, and evaluating outcomes. The simulation scenario student learning outcomes on Part 1 of the Clinical Simulation Scenario Template (Chapter 4) are paired with the CJMM competencies. To measure specific student learning, expected behaviors are written for every step in the scenario and linked to the relevant competency. Below is the scenario for patient Jonathan Farmer and the student performance behaviors for the scenario.

Scenario

Patient Name: Jonathan Farmer **Age:** 45 **WT:** 84 KG
Dx: Open Left Tib/Fib Fracture with Open Reduction Internal Fixation repair, T1 Burst Fracture, Liver Laceration, Rheumatoid Arthritis
Lines & Tubes: Left Triple Lumen, PEG, Art Line **IV Fluids:** NS at 125 mL/hr, Almost empty Fresh Frozen Plasma hanging, PCA Pump Orders
Drips: None **Allergies:** NKA **Needed for Scenario:** Left leg wound, C-Collar, FFP, Signed Surgery and Blood Consents, Blank Preop Checklist

Scenario Progression

DOB: 08-08-1980

Student Actions Student Performance Behaviors	**Mannequin Response Faculty (Health Care Provider) Communication**
- Checks MD orders - Verifies IV pumps working and correct fluids hanging, verifies PCA pump orders - Reverse T-Berg - Puts side rails up - Introduces themselves - Checks patient name and birthdate →	**Opening Vital Signs on Monitor:** **Heart rhythm: NSR HR: 120** **ABP: 152/88 RR: 24 SaO2: 95%** **Temp: Periph 99.9** **Breath Sounds: Rhonchi**
- Takes down 1st unit FFP and calls BB for second one - Assesses Pain → - Gives RN Bolus via PCA ← - Evaluates response → - Changes left leg dressing - Gives PEG meds and SQ meds	"Jonathan Farmer, 8-8-80" "In pain for last 2 hours; it's an 8." HR 90 128/72 16 "That helped."

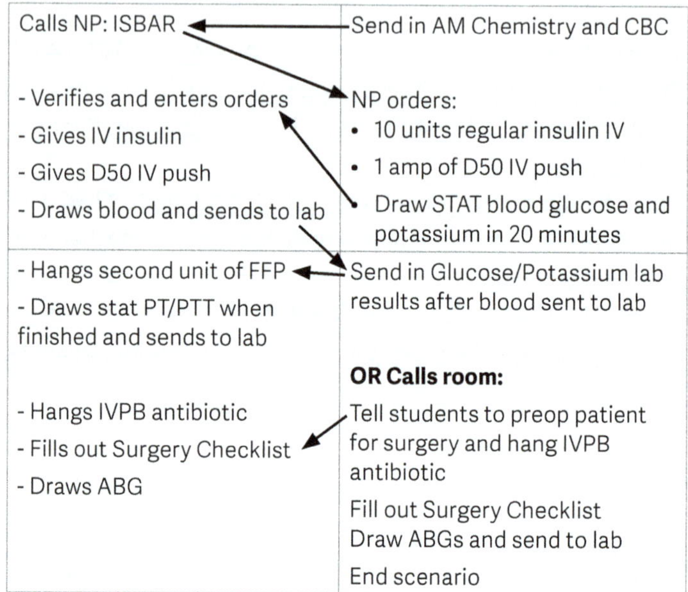

Calls NP: ISBAR	Send in AM Chemistry and CBC
- Verifies and enters orders - Gives IV insulin - Gives D50 IV push - Draws blood and sends to lab	NP orders: • 10 units regular insulin IV • 1 amp of D50 IV push • Draw STAT blood glucose and potassium in 20 minutes
- Hangs second unit of FFP - Draws stat PT/PTT when finished and sends to lab - Hangs IVPB antibiotic - Fills out Surgery Checklist - Draws ABG	Send in Glucose/Potassium lab results after blood sent to lab **OR Calls room:** Tell students to preop patient for surgery and hang IVPB antibiotic Fill out Surgery Checklist Draw ABGs and send to lab End scenario

Lab results sent into room:

Lab results: Jonathan Farmer **Pt ID:** 00003 **DOB:** 08-08-1980
Specimen collected: Admission Day 0600 **Specimen:** Blood, Fasting

Test Name	Patient Results	Reference Range
BMP:		
Sodium	**136**	135–145 mEq/L
Potassium	**6.2***	3.5–5.0 mEq/L
Chloride	**105**	98–108 mEq/L
Calcium	**9.0**	8.6–10.6 mEq/L
Albumin	**4.0**	3.2–5 g/dL
BUN	**22**	7–23 mg/dL
Creatinine	**1.5**	.7–1.7 mg/dL
Glucose	**75**	70–110 mg/dL
Misc Chem:		

CPK	**25,000***	22–198 u/L
CBC:		
WBC	**13***	3.5-11 x109/L
Hemoglobin	**12**	13-18 g/dL
Hematocrit	**50**	45-62%

Student Performance Behaviors

Type of Sim: CC **Faculty:** __________ **Date:** ______________

Patient Name: Jonathan Farmer **Age:** 8-8-1980 45 **WT:** 84KG

Dx: Open Left Tib/Fib Fracture with Open Reduction Internal Fixation repair, T1 Burst Fracture, Liver Laceration, Rheumatoid Arthritis

Lines & Tubes: Left Triple Lumen, PEG, Art Line

IV Fluids: NS at 125 mL/hr, Almost empty Fresh Frozen Plasma, Second bag of FFP **Drips:** none **Allergies:** _____ NKA _____

Needed for Scenario: Left leg wound, C-Collar, Fresh Frozen Plasma, Signed Surgery and Blood Consents, Blank Preop Checklist ______________________

Beginning Vital Signs:

Heart rhythm: ST 120 **ABP:** 152/88 **RR:** 24 **SaO2:** 95%

Temp: 99.9 **Breath Sounds:** Decreased

STUDENT PERFORMANCE BEHAVIORS	OBSERVED SPBs : Y or N	CJM LAYERS
Checks MD orders		SAFETY-Retention of Learning Measurement
Verifies IV pumps working and correct fluids hanging		SAFETY-Retention of Learning Measurement
Patient placed in 30 degrees reverse Trendelenburg		SAFETY-Retention of Learning Measurement

Puts side rails up		SAFETY-Retention of Learning Measurement
Introduces themselves		SAFETY-Retention of Learning Measurement
Performs head-to-toe assessment		SAFETY-Retention of Learning Measurement
Checks patient name and birthdate "Response = Johnathan Farmer"		SAFETY-Retention of Learning Measurement
Asks if in pain "Response = Yes" Bolus via PCA Reassess for pain		CHS - ACTION SAFETY-Retention of Learning Measurement EVAL
Takes down 1st unit FFP and calls BB for second one		CHS - ACTION
Send in second unit FFP and AM Chemistry and CBC Test Results		
Calls NP with High K: ID self ISBAR Gives current problem: • Vital signs, labs, assessment data Offers recommendation Repeats orders		RA CUES, H-S ACTION
NP Orders: 10 Units Regular Insulin IVP, 1 amp D50 IVP, Draw STAT blood glucose and potassium level in 20 minutes		
Verifies and enters orders Gives IV Insulin Gives D50 IVP Draws blood from arterial line and sends to lab Rechecks blood glucose with glucometer		ACTION, SAFETY-Retention of Learning ACTION, SKILLS/SAFETY-Retention of Learning ACTION, SKILLS/SAFETY-Retention of Learning ACTION, SKILLS/SAFETY-Retention of Learning EVAL

Hangs second unit of FFP Draws STAT PT/ PTT when finished		CHS-ACTION SKILLS/SAFETY-Retention of Learning
Changes left leg dressing using sterile technique		CHS-ACTION SKILLS/SAFETY-Retention of Learning
Call room: Tell to preop patient for surgery and hang antibiotic Fill out preop checklist Draw ABGs and send to lab		
Hangs IVPB correctly		ACTION, SKILLS/ SAFETY-Retention of Learning
Fills out Surgery Checklist		ACTION, SKILLS/ SAFETY-Retention of Learning
Draws ABGs correctly		ACTION, SKILLS/ SAFETY-Retention of Learning

SAFETY can include anything you want, especially program safety SPBs.

SKILLS/SAFETY identifies skills they should be able to perform that are also important to safety because if they do them wrong it endangers the patient.

RETENTION OF LEARNING is when a psychomotor skill is performed correctly.

R/A CUES, H-S (recognize/analyze cues, hypothesis-solution) is any cue they are given (like vital signs, lab results, physical assessment, things the mother says, things the patient says) that they identify needs to be reported to an NP.

ACTION is when the NP is contacted and the intervention they ordered is carried out.

CHS-ACTION is when a cue is noted and the student independently performs action from standing orders (sliding scale insulin, pain medications).

EVAL is when a patient evaluation is performed.

Student Evaluation

The results are used during debriefing and for follow-up with the student's clinical faculty. If the clinical performance of the student was weak in certain areas, the clinical faculty can refocus the student on mastering the skill. If a student is struggling in clinical and in simulation, this data is used in the need for a performance improvement plan.

Course Evaluation

The design of the junior- and senior-level simulations includes that each student attend two different simulation days. The first simulation day (SIM 1) involves two scenarios (4 students each) caring for low- to medium-acuity patients after they have started their clinical rotation. The second simulation day (SIM 2) also has two scenarios but with a higher acuity and occurs toward the end of the semester. The number of times the scenario runs is determined by how many students are in the class that semester. Then for each behavior, the percentage of correct times it was performed during the semester is determined by adding the number of correct divided by the number of times it was run. If you run Jonathan Farmer on 10 days, there will be 10 Student Performance Behavior sheets for Mr. Farmer. The percentage of each SPB on the sheet is determined by dividing the number of correct times out of 10 that occurred divided by 10 and then times 100 to give the percentage. If the SPB of checking two methods of patient ID was correctly performed on 6 forms, you would take 6 divided by 10, which is .6, multiplied by 100%, which gives you a 60% correct performance of the SPB. The pass rate for the school of nursing is used to determine the pass rate for SPBs. For example, if the school passes students whose final grade in a course is 75%, an SPB performed correctly for the semester 75% of the attempts is considered acceptable for that particular SPB. The 60% correct performance of identifying patients by two methods would be considered unacceptable performance for the nursing program and would require a plan for improvement, as this is a program safety SPB. This data is used as part of the annual school assessment plan and the end-of-semester course report.

Program Evaluation

The safety and communication SPBs are part of every scenario. Therefore, the results for these SPBs are combined for all scenarios in the semester. The percentage for each safety and communication SPB in all scenarios that were performed correctly is determined. If any SPB falls below the passing rate, it is scrutinized closer for a possible reason. The correction is usually to take a different approach in teaching the importance of the safety and communication SPBs with the sophomore class and continue through the junior and senior years. This feedback loop is used as part of the accreditation process, both for the specific nursing accreditation entity and the university accrediting bodies. Data that is consistently above the passing percentage is used as a measure of acceptable end-of-program performance.

Determination of the Outcome of Simulation SPBs With the Integration of the CJMM

The CJMM uses three layers to demonstrate the six actions students use to devise clinical judgments (see Chapter 1). These six cognitive processes are measurable and define how nurses learn clinical judgment over time:

1. Recognize cues.
2. Analyze cues.
3. Prioritize hypotheses.
4. Generate solutions.
5. Take action.
6. Evaluate outcomes.

SPBs were developed for each of the six cognitive processes and used to form a data collection sheet for nursing student actions. The correct performance of each SPB by the student determined the patient's outcome. The outcomes were determined and presented in a poster format at the American Association of College of Nurses annual conference.

Evaluation of Integrating the CJMM into Clinical Simulation to Improve Student Performance Behaviors in Patient Rescue Scenarios

Purpose: The purpose of these complex scenarios was to use the model of clinical judgment and decision-making abilities to promote nursing recognition and appropriate responses with a deteriorating patient.

Processes/Procedures: Groups of 4–5 senior-level students cared for one critically ill patient in Sim 1 and in Sim 2 as a team. Each student attended both simulation days but only cared for one patient each day. Sim 1 was basic; Sim 2 had a higher acuity. All simulations lasted 1–2 hours with medications, recognizing/analyzing cues for problems, prioritizing hypotheses, calling an NP, taking actions, and evaluating outcomes. Each scenario had specific student performance behaviors (SPBs) for each of the following cognitive operations:

- R/A CUES, H-S (recognize/analyze cues, hypothesis-solution) was any cue they were given (like vital signs, lab results, physical assessment, things the mother said, things the patient said) that they identify needed to be reported to an NP.
- ACTION was when the NP was contacted and the intervention they ordered was carried out.
- CHS-ACTION was when a cue was noted and the student independently performed action from standing orders (sliding scale insulin, pain medications).
- EVAL was when a patient evaluation was performed.

The CJMM was incorporated into simulation at the senior level in 2020.

Results: To determine the impact of focusing SPBs on the CJMM layers, data on SPB performance from 1 year before introducing the CJMM (2019) was compared to SPB performance for 2 years after the model was introduced into simulation (2020–2021). The actual results of the data are included in the charts below.

This data is for senior students only. SIM 1 was a basic admission scenario into an ICU, and SIM 2 was a complex admission scenario involving a ventilator and advanced cardiac monitoring.

Three Years of Simulation Data

From 2019 to 2021, both Sim 1 and Sim 2 had 10 cognitive operations in every scenario. Data was collected over 3 years.

75% Performance Is Considered Passing

SAFETY

- SIM 1 and SIM 2: All SPBs are >75% for all years
- In SIM 2, improvement with recognizing that HOB elevated is wrong action for hypotension

SAFETY: Can include anything you want to include in your safety monitoring

- All SPBs are >75% for all years
- Improvement with recognizing that HOB elevated is wrong action with hypotension
- All SPBs are >75% for all years
- Improvement with recognizing that HOB elevated is wrong action with hypotension

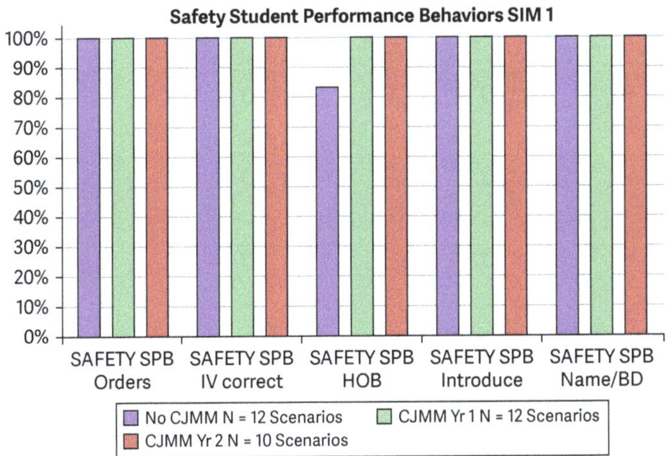

FIGURE 5.1 Safety Student Performance Behaviors: SIM 1

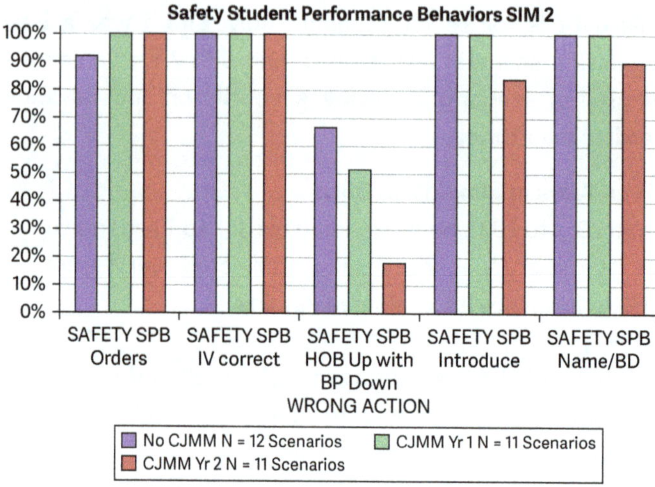

FIGURE 5.2 Safety Student Performance Behaviors: SIM 2

SKILLS/SAFETY: Identifies skills they should be able to perform that are also safety because if they do them wrong it endangers the patient

SIM 1

- All skills performed correctly and safely except for IVPB, which was < 75% until CJMM Yr 2 when it was >75%

SIM 2

- All skills safe > 75%

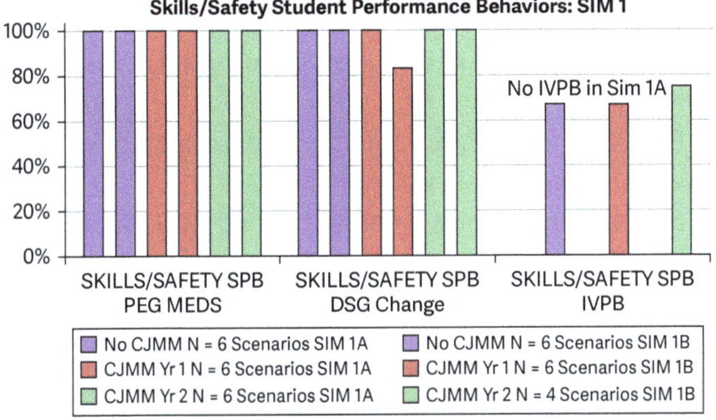

FIGURE 5.3 Skills/Safety Student Performance Behaviors: SIM 1

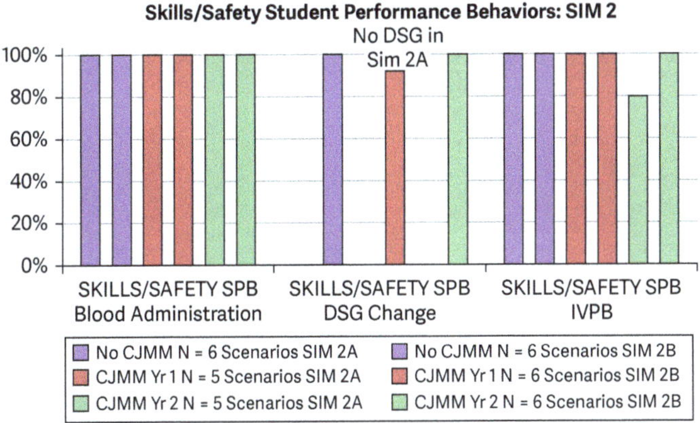

FIGURE 5.4 Skills/Safety Student Performance Behaviors: SIM 2

CHS-A: When a cue is noted, a hypothesis is generated, a solution is decided upon, and the student independently and correctly performs an action using preordered interventions or their knowledge base

SIM 1: Patient 1A & Patient 1B

- All SPB for glucose monitoring and use of SSI to administer insulin are >75%
- SPB of pain assessment and treatment with a PCA bolus below 75% for CJMM Yr 1
- SPB of evaluation of pain <75% in No CJMM, 100% CJMM

SIM 2: Patient A

- SPB of using admission order to increase infusing vasopressor with hypotension <75% in CJMM Yr 2
- SPB of using admission order to send ABG for low SpO2 <75% CJMM Yr 1

R/A CUES, HS/ACTION:

Any cue (like vital signs, lab results, physical assessment, comments by patient/family) that student hypothesizes needs intervention by an NP

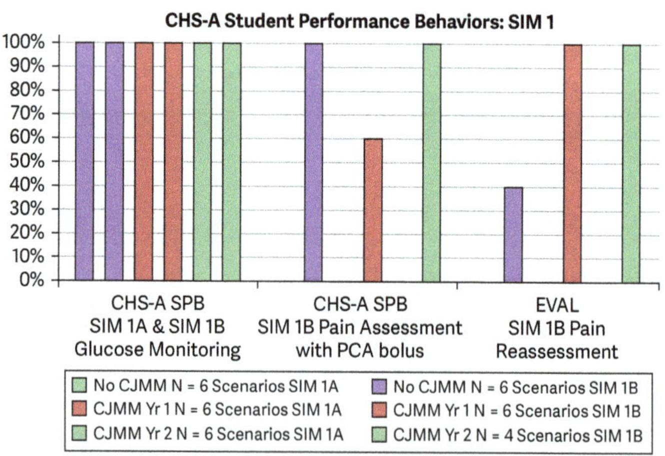

FIGURE 5.5 CHS-A Student Performance Behaviors: SIM 1

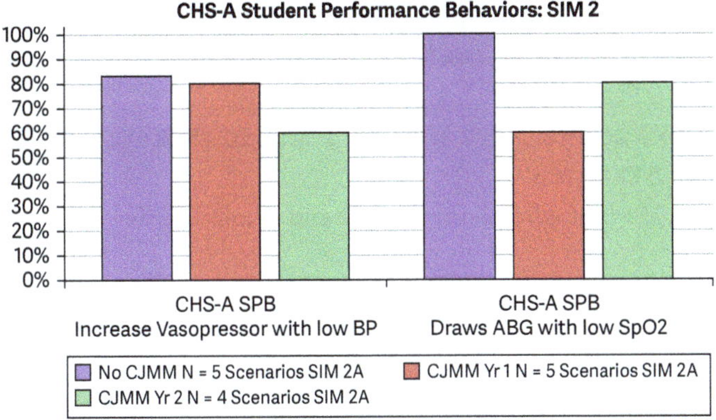

FIGURE 5.6 CHS-A Student Performance Behaviors: SIM 2

SIM 1: Patient 1A & Patient 1B

- All SPB >75% for call NP with abnormal lab

SIM 1: Patient A

- SPB of K Run <75% in CJMM Yr 1, up to 100% in CJMM Yr 2

SIM 1: Patient B

- All SPB of administering D50 and insulin >75%

SIM 2: Patient A

- All SPB >75% for call to NP for hypotension
- SPB of hanging second vasopressor <75% in No CJMM, >75% in CJMM Yrs 1 & 2
- SPB of vent changes <75% in CJMM Yr 1
- All SPB of evaluation by drawing ABG <75%
- SPB of wrong action with hypotension 60% in No CJMM, decreased to 30% in CJMM Yr 2

SIM 2: Patient B

- All SPB >75% for call NP with critical lab

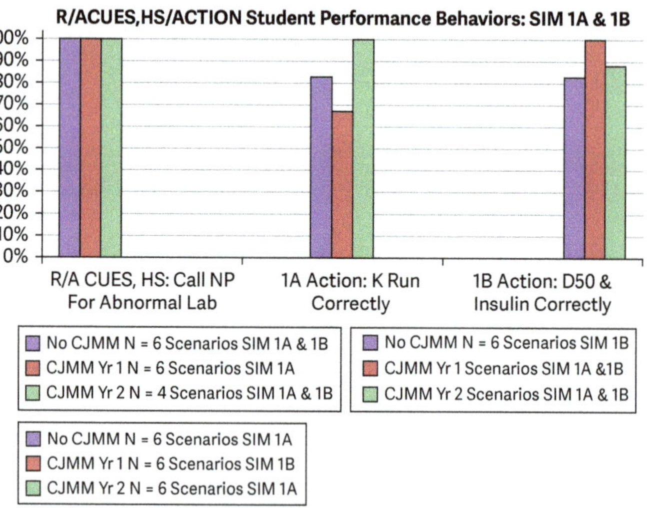

FIGURE 5.7 R/A CUES, HS/ACTION Student Performance Behaviors: SIM 1A & 1B

- All SPB >75% for hanging Insulin drip
- SPB for calling NP due to hypotension <75% in 2019
- All SPB > 75% for hanging RBCs correctly

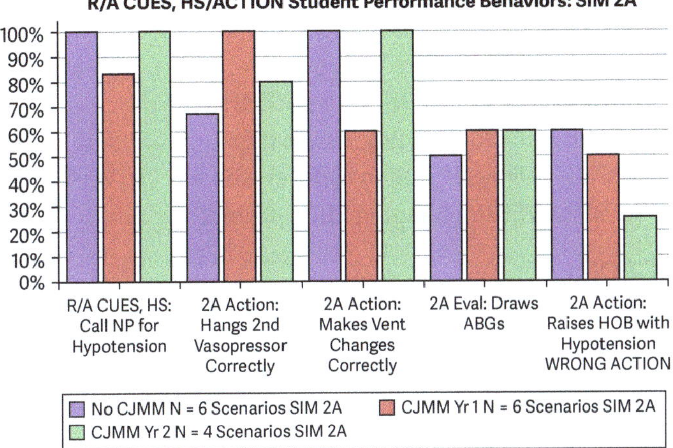

FIGURE 5.8 R/A CUES, HS/ACTION Student Performance Behaviors: SIM 2A

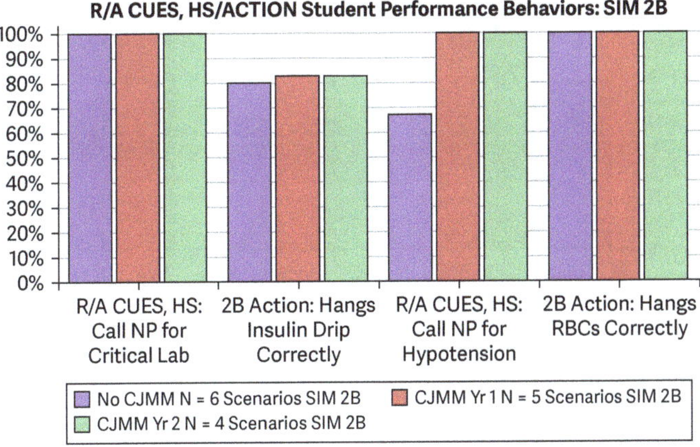

FIGURE 5.9 R/A CUES, HS/ACTION Student Performance Behaviors: SIM 2B

ACTION then EVAL

SIM 1A

- SPB for heparin bolus <75% in No CJMM, >75% in CJMM years
- SPB for heparin drip <75% in No CJMM, >75% in CJMM years
- All EVAL >75%

SIM 2B

- All SPB >75% for call NP with critical lab
- All SPB >75% for hanging insulin drip
- SPB for calling NP due to hypotension <75% in No CJMM
- All SPB > 75% for hanging RBCs correctly

ACTION:

The NP is contacted and the intervention they ordered is carried out correctly

EVAL:

(Evaluation) An action that results in the effectiveness of an intervention

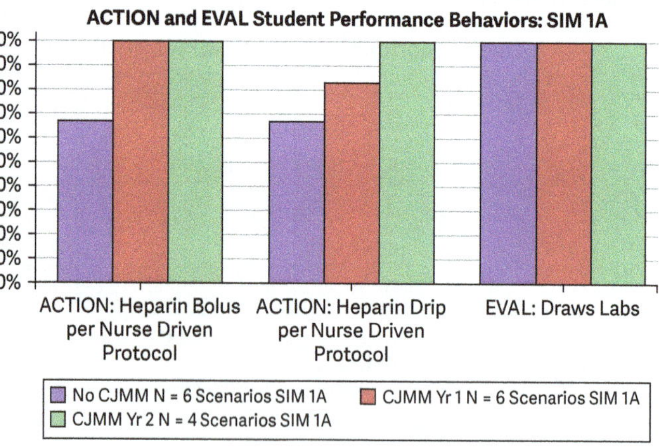

FIGURE 5.10 ACTION and EVAL Student Performance Behaviors: SIM 1A

Conclusions/Implications for Practice: Incorporating the CJMM into a complex team-based simulation focused on rescuing patients increases correct student performance of the model's cognitive operations.

Source: Mcilvoy, L., & McMahan, J. (2022, December, 1–3). Transformation of simulation that connects the CJMM to patient rescue scenarios improving student performance behaviors [Poster presentation]. American Association of Colleges of Nursing, Chicago, IL, United States. https://www.aacnnursing.org/transform/past-presentations

Summary

Data demonstrates that the safety SPBs were consistently above the pass rate. This can be attributed to the use of the same safety SPBs from sophomore through senior simulations. The concept of perfusion and HOB position was clearly misunderstood as represented by the data. To remedy this, the pathophysiology of what occurs with perfusion during HOB manipulation was reinforced during didactic. All skills except IV piggyback administration were consistently acceptable. This is due to the redesign of the sophomore foundations course into a simulation experience with students producing mastery videos for the seven most complex skills (see Chapter 2). At the beginning of the simulation program, only 50% of senior students could perform skills correctly. The model of deliberate practice and the CJMM provided consistent methods for helping students retain proficiency in psychomotor skill performance, recognize the cues of patient deterioration, and determine which actions rescue their patient. Changes in classrooms, clinical settings, and simulations should be driven by data. Using these models provides data that can be used to determine if the mode and content of the educational experience are effective in terms of student performance behaviors.

References

Mcilvoy, L., & McMahan, J. (2022, December, 1–3). *Transformation of simulation that connects the CJMM to patient rescue scenarios improving student performance behaviors* [poster presentation]. American Association of Colleges of Nursing, Chicago, IL, United States. https://www.aacnnursing.org/transform/past-presentations

National Institutes of Health Office of Human Resources. (n.d.). *What are competencies?* Retrieved May 11, 2024, from https://hr.nih.gov/about/faq/working-nih/competencies/what-are-competencies

CHAPTER 6

The Logistics of Starting/Maintaining Clinical Simulation

Learning Outcomes

- Recognize the need for adequate space and equipment for simulation.
- Secure financing as needed for both durable and expendable equipment.
- Develop methods to collect data on simulation outcomes.
- Share simulation techniques and student outcomes via presentations/publications.

The Physical Lab

Most schools of nursing have an area that is used as a lab that contains the basic equipment to teach students psychomotor skills (e.g., hospital beds, blood pressure equipment, IV equipment, etc.). This area can also be used for simulation. Having faculty in the same room during simulation is how many simulation labs started. There are also portable two-way mirrors that can be used with faculty in the same room. A mannequin that has no extras for skills training can be used for simulation when you add the necessary props for realistic skill performance (see Chapter 7). You can also use skill trainers and add what is missing for clinical simulation.

If you want a bedside monitor that shows realistic vital signs that you can alter as the scenario progresses, you can download computer programs or apps that will load onto phones and pads, both apple and android. Search simulated vital signs app to see a variety of products. The ability to alter vital signs and EKG rhythms during a scenario enhances the ability to provide a realistic experience for students. Prices and functionality for these programs are variable, as some only provide vital signs with no EKG rhythm, while others allow you to program what is seen on the screen to enable the use of sophisticated monitoring variables, such as central venous pressure and pulmonary artery pressure measurements. Chapter 7 demonstrates how to include the realistic use of this level of monitoring. Some of the newer skills mannequins are equipped with programmable bedside monitors. If you have a mannequin that comes with a bedside monitor, you can use this monitor with any other mannequin by using its computer controller.

Financing Simulation Mannequins and Durable/Expendable Equipment

There are several methods of securing financing for durable and expendable mannequins and lab equipment. Securing a grant is one of the most common sources of simulation funds. Research grants are offered from federal, state, and local government entities, universities, hospitals, and national nursing organizations. Many have very specific requirements for eligibility, which makes it difficult for smaller schools of nursing to acquire such a grant. However, most foundation grants are available to local groups whose aim is to improve the conditions for members of the community. Both are reviewed below.

Research Grants

The associations that support simulation (see Chapter 1) offer research grants.

INACSL: The Debra Spunt Research Grant funds research that advances simulation in healthcare.

https://www.inacsl.org/index.php?option=com_content&view=article&id=91:debra-spunt-research-grant&catid=20:site-content

SSH: The Early Career Simulation Research Grant Program supports the development of new investigators and their research initiatives.

https://www.ssih.org/About-SSH/Development/Early-Career-Research-Grant-Program

National League of Nursing (NLN): Four to five grants are awarded annually that meet their priorities for research. Simulation research meets their objective of connecting the science of nursing education with the science of learning.

https://www.nln.org/education/grants-scholarships/professional-development-programsgrants-and-scholarships/nln-nursing-education-research-grants-program

Foundation Grants

There are several kinds of foundation grants. Every state in the United States has counties (though Louisiana calls its counties "parishes" and Alaska uses "boroughs"). There are over 700 county-based community foundations in the United States. The mission of these foundations is to provide funding for projects and programs that will benefit the community they represent. School of nursing faculty can apply for this funding, as the aim of simulation is to improve the knowledge and performance of nursing graduates who take jobs within the community, thereby improving the health of the community. Each of these county foundations will have a website that explains their funding process. Awards range from $200 to $20,000 depending on the county. Some have scheduled awards, and others let community members request grants as needed. County foundations have individuals who fund some of their grants. An ideal first step would be to have the dean of the school of nursing contact them to ask if they have philanthropists who are interested in partnering with a local school of nursing to improve the health of the community. This type of donor may be interested in financing a mannequin that would exceed the amount the community foundation is capable of awarding.

Another foundation source of funding is casinos. Many casinos have foundations that offer grants similar to the county foundations. Some casinos are mandated to offer foundation grants as part of their licensing agreement with the county. The grants may or may not be restricted to the county where they are located. They also have websites that offer explanations for applying for a grant. Table 6.1 contains a list of states with non-tribal casinos and states with tribal casinos.

TABLE 6.1

States With Non-Tribal Casinos		States With Tribal Casinos
Arkansas	Nevada	California
Colorado	New Jersey	Connecticut
Illinois	New York	Florida
Indiana	Ohio	Idaho
Iowa	Pennsylvania	Indiana
Kansas	Rhode Island	Minnesota
Louisiana	South Dakota	New York
Maine	Virginia	Oklahoma
Maryland	West Virginia	South Dakota
Massachusetts		Wyoming
Michigan		

Foundation grants are written in simple language that explains why the money is needed and exactly how the money will be spent. A template of topics that need to be addressed are usually supplied in the application process. Most high-value financial grants require that the community organization match their spending to the amount of grant money that is being requested. The following textbox contains an example of an actual community foundation grant from a casino that was awarded $20,000.

After receiving a large grant, it is important that the donor is recognized by plaques outside the door and a full demonstration of a simulation using the equipment that they financed. This encourages continual support and strengthens feelings of appreciation in all parties.

Casino Grant Application Example

A. Project need

1. **Project description**

Educating student nurses requires that they practice nursing skills on real people. These clinical experiences occur frequently in hospitals and involve the use of a lot of faculty and hospital resources. Clinical simulation was developed to offer students an alternative clinical learning experience. In clinical simulation, students enter a hospital room and are presented with an adult or pediatric reality-based mannequin that has a history, diagnosis, and medication orders just like the real-world patient. Only in clinical simulation can the student take time to critically think about which actions are appropriate, and they have the luxury of making mistakes (and learning from them) without harm. In 2007, the School of Nursing bought its first adult simulation mannequin (the SIMMAN™ for $39,388) and piloted a plan to integrate it into the clinical experiences of senior nursing students during the class that focuses on the care of patients in the intensive care unit (ICU). Caring for these very ill and complex patients is incredibly stressful for nursing students. To be exposed to an ICU setting in clinical simulation first would allow them to practice in a less stressful, safer environment.

Initially, the SIMMAN was placed in an empty lab room and faculty developed beginning clinical scenarios that all 50 students went through individually and advanced scenarios that involved groups of 3–5 students problem-solving multiple issues. Student evaluations of this pilot program rated their experiences as very positive; 100% agreed on a standardized evaluation form that they developed the ability to solve actual problems, develop needed skills, and were exposed to a variety of clinical problems. To expand our use of clinical simulation into junior-year clinicals, pediatric and infant simulation mannequins were purchased ($6,146). In the summer of 2008, we will reconstruct the nursing lab to open a second simulation hospital room to house the pediatric/infant mannequins for $8,500.

The greater the reality of the simulated hospital room, the easier it is for students to react realistically to clinical scenarios. The original adult room was quickly outfitted with the essentials needed, and there is no equipment yet for the pediatric/infant hospital room. This grant will be used to purchase durable medical equipment, such as simulated oxygen and suction panels for the walls, IV and feeding pumps, medication and crash carts, and a ventilator. Expendable equipment needed for the first year will also be purchased and thereafter incorporated into the School of Nursing's budget.

2. **Problems addressed**

   During the pilot simulation experiences, the instructor taped an oxygen flow meter to the wall and had students place a sticky note with how much oxygen the student wanted delivered to the flow meter. Inexpensive plastic carts were used for medication carts, and there were no working IV or feeding pumps. The instructor was in the room with the student and SIMMAN™ operating the computer that controls the SIMMAN™. The SIMMAN™ is a very realistic mannequin that is anatomically correct for either sex, has heart, lung, and bowel sounds, can receive any type of medication, can have any kind of tube inserted, including a breathing tube or a tracheostomy, and is able to have a conversation with the student. With the appropriate realistic hospital equipment, a credible hospital environment can be created making it easier for the students to readily accept the reality of the simulation and perform accordingly. After the construction, the instructor will be in an adjoining room observing the student through a two-way mirror. This will reinforce the reality of being alone with a patient and reacting to events as they occur.

3. **Project timeline**

   The adult SIMMAN and the pediatric and infant mannequins have been purchased using university money. The SIMMAN pilot project is complete and will now move into a formal research stage where the instructor will formally investigate the impact clinical simulation has on critical thinking skills of senior nursing students. The pilot phase of using the pediatric/infant mannequins with the junior-level nursing students is underway this semester. Summer of 2008 the university will reconstruct the nursing lab so that there will be both adult and pediatric/infant hospital rooms with an observation room between them from which the instructors can operate the mannequins and observe the students. During the summer of 2008 the durable and expendable medical equipment will be purchased with the foundation grant money from reliable medical supply companies via the internet. August of 2008 both rooms will be outfitted with the purchased medical equipment by the nursing faculty. September of 2008 both rooms will officially be opened with a reception and demonstrations of clinical simulations.

B. Project impact

1. **Project accomplishments**

   Furnishing the clinical simulation hospital rooms with realistic equipment will enhance the reality of all of our clinical simulations. The closer to real-world the environment is, the more apt students are to react exactly how they would in a hospital situation. As we continue to incorporate clinical simulation into our curriculum, strengthening the reality of the environment in which the clinical simulations take place will make it easier to incorporate clinical simulations into more sophomore- and junior-level classes in which their exposure to hospital environments is still limited. The more alike the clinical simulation hospital rooms are to actual hospital rooms, the easier it will be to successfully transition these students into hospital clinical experiences.

2. **Project evaluation**
   Both simulation hospital rooms will be equipped with the new equipment and functional by fall semester 2008. The adult SIMMAN room will be used with senior nursing students fall semester 2008 in their intensive care class and with sophomore students learning basic health assessment skills (listening to normal heart and lung sounds). The pediatric/infant simulation room will be used with junior and sophomore students fall semester 2008 to learn both basic and advanced health assessment skills on this age group. Spring semester 2009 the junior students will be exposed to basic clinical scenarios in groups to begin to teach them clinical decision-making skills. Standard evaluation forms will be given to all students seeking their opinion on whether clinical simulation allowed them to develop the ability to solve actual problems, develop needed skills, and if they felt they were exposed to a variety of clinical problems
3. **Project benefit to the county**
   The School of Nursing uses the local hospital and health services as a major clinical site. Using clinical simulation to prepare our nursing students for their hospital clinical experience will enhance their ability to provide competent and safe care to the citizens of the county. In addition, a large number of our graduate nurses seek employment at the hospital. The stronger their clinical preparation as a nurse is, the more proficient they will be in their nursing care of the citizens of the county.

Equipment

To gain access to expendable equipment (e.g., syringes, IV tubing, dressing supplies, etc.), look for companies that have partnered with local hospitals to receive medical/nursing equipment that can no longer be used within their facility because it is expired. This equipment is still functioning and often in its sterile packaging. These nonprofit organizations send vital medical equipment that is still working overseas to healthcare providers and facilities but cannot send expired equipment. Most are glad to partner with nursing schools and provide them with a large variety of nursing equipment and supplies, such as dressing supplies, needles, syringes, IV equipment, drainage tubes and bags, lab supplies, and more. Partner with these organizations, such as SOS International, to receive the equipment that cannot be sent overseas. Look on social media for SOS-sponsored sites and other organizations that have access to expired healthcare equipment. Use your school's social media presence to ask the community to consider donating unused healthcare supplies that are open and/or expired. Urinary catheterization and tracheal suctioning kits are common supplies that families have after a loved one passes. Occasionally the Goodwill will receive medical supplies that they cannot sell and might donate to a School of Nursing or sell at a very low price.

Another idea is to go to the Chief Nursing Officers of all the local hospitals and discuss partnering with the hospital to take all their expired equipment and supplies for use in the simulation lab. Supply them with bins to be placed on units throughout the hospital where the staff can place expired equipment. Set up a collection and pickup process. Advertise your collection process throughout the hospitals to ensure that the appropriate equipment is donated. Contact the Operating Room and Post Anesthesia Care Unit, as they end up with the most expired equipment.

Dissemination of Simulation Techniques and Outcomes

Most publications and presentations on simulation are done by larger programs with designated simulation faculty, yet the successes and failures of smaller programs need to be shared. It is important that all simulation faculty take the step toward presenting the details of their program. It starts with collecting data. Using student performance behaviors, or whatever you wish to call them, faculty need to collect data on individual student performance and course performance of psychomotor skills, patient safety, and clinical judgment. This data drives program assessment and course improvement. This data is also helpful in presenting what your simulation program does and how you do it.

Beginning presenters are more comfortable presenting in poster formats rather than podium presentations, which is what most accomplished presenters do. But both modalities require the same abstracts that are used to decide who is accepted to present. The first step in applying to present is to go to the call for abstracts website. Most national conferences have websites that you have to set up with a username and password. Within this site you will enter all of your contact information, including your CV and your bio that is relevant to your abstract topic (see below). The specifics of the abstract will be there. There is a word or character limit for both the title of the abstract and the body of the abstract. The objectives of the conference will be stated. It is advantageous if you can link your abstract title to an objective, such as using the same terminology.

The next step is to write the abstract. An *abstract* is a summary of the project that includes the importance of the project (why it matters), what you specifically did in the project, and what the results or impact of the project were. First write one or two sentences that explain why the topic is important. Next describe what you specifically did during the project. Then discuss the findings or impact of the project. End with a sentence summarizing what the poster will present. Some organizations want a teaching plan. Below is an accepted national abstract for a poster and the teaching plan.

From Conference Brochure Poster Session Objectives:

- Explore strategies to integrate technology into curriculum and practice.
- Discuss current best practice for education and research.
- Identify creative solutions for enhancing utilization of Simulation/Skills lab.

Abstract

Incorporating Student Simulation Outcomes Into a School of Nursing Plan for Assessment of Student Learning

National accreditation of schools of nursing requires that teaching-learning practices be self-evaluated to foster ongoing program improvements. To this aim, a Midwestern BSN program incorporated senior-level student simulation outcomes into their annual Plan for Assessment of Student Learning. The assessment plan is based on nine school of nursing program outcomes and their corresponding measurable competencies. The results of this continuous assessment plan are discussed with all faculty annually, and a plan of action is determined. All clinical simulation scenarios within the school of nursing program have evidence-based student performance objectives. These student performance objectives have been evaluated by the same faculty that developed the scenarios since their inception. Data on achievement of specific simulation objectives was incorporated into the assessment plan under the appropriate student competency. In the beginning years, data demonstrated that many psychomotor skills that were taught and supposedly mastered as part of the sophomore-level fundamentals course were not performed competently by senior students. In 2012, using the feedback loop and based on our data, we derived an action plan where we would modify our sophomore-level fundamentals course into a clinical simulation experience. Every year we collect and analyze data on student performance objective achievement and derive a plan based upon the results. This poster will present the Plan for Assessment of Student Learning, the student simulation outcomes incorporated into the plan, and the details of the annual action plans for program improvement that have been developed and incorporated using longitudinal student simulation data.

Education Planning Table

Title of Activity: Incorporating Student Simulation Outcomes Into a School of Nursing Plan for Assessment of Student Learning

Identified Gap(s): Knowledge of utilizing simulation for program assessment

Description of current state: Faculty are well versed in writing course objectives/outcomes

Description of desired/achievable state: Recognition that each course has a role in achieving program outcomes and recognition that simulation can be used to measure program outcomes and competencies

Gap to be addressed by this activity:

x Knowledge _____ Skills x Practice _____ Other

Learning Outcome (select all that apply): x Nursing Professional Development ☐ Patient Outcome ☐ Other: Describe **1. Identify components of a Plan of Assessment for student learning outcomes** **2. Determine how to incorporate student simulation outcomes into Program Assessment** **3. Discuss implementation of the feedback loop using student simulation outcome data to direct Program Improvement**			
CONTENT (Topics)	**TIME FRAME (if live)**	**PRESENTER/ AUTHOR**	**TEACHING METHODS/ LEARNER ENGAGEMENT STRATEGIES**
Provide an outline of the content below to align with learning outcomes listed above.	Exact time required for content	L. Mcilvoy	Reading Poster, Discussion
1. Example of a Plan of Assessment with measurable student competencies		L. Mcilvoy	Reading Poster, Discussion

2. Presentation of student simulation outcomes that are used as the measurable tool for student competencies		L. McIlvoy	Reading Poster, Discussion
3. Diagram of feedback loop that explains how to use student simulation outcome data to change curriculum and direct program improvement		L. McIlvoy	Reading Poster, Discussion
List the evidence-based references used for developing this educational activity: Commission on Collegiate Nursing Education. (2013). *Standards for accreditation of baccalaureate and graduate nursing programs.* Jeffries, P. (2009). A framework for designing, implementing, and educating simulations used as teaching strategies. *Nursing Education Perspectives, 26*, 96–103. American Association of Higher Education. (1996). *Nine principles of good practice for assessing student learning.* https://www.ncat.edu/_files/pdfs/campus-life/nine-principles.pdf			

Source: McIlvoy, L., & McMahan, J. (2017, June 22–24). Incorporating student simulation outcomes into a school of nursing plan for assessment of student learning *[poster presentation]. International Nursing Association of Clinical Simulation and Learning Conference, Washington, DC, United States.*

Summary

Clinical simulation requires significant time and money. However, as an educational technique, it is priceless. Nurses have always been master problem-solvers. We are creative, resourceful, and frequently inspired. Acquiring financial support is a challenge with many possible solutions. When clinical simulation is explained to members of the community, they instantly see the educational value. We need to communicate our ingenuity in using simulation as an educational technique—for the advancement of our profession and our careers.

CHAPTER 7

The Magic of the Reality Behind Simulation

Learning Outcomes

- Prepare mannequins to replicate the reality of the setting that is to be used in each scenario.
- Build intravenous (IV) lines (peripheral, triple lumens, percutaneous intravenous central catheter [PICC], and introducer sheaths) that are capable of having fluids and blood products infused.
- Create a simulated blood supply to use where real blood would be necessary.

Simulation that is enhanced with working intravenous lines of all kinds, a bedside monitor that provides vital signs, wounds that appear realistic, and the ability to realistically administer all routes of medications allows students to accept the premise that they are caring for a real patient in a true scenario. The equipment needed and the process of assembling pieces to create a functioning item will be demonstrated in this chapter. The particular brands on the pieces are not important, just their function.

Intravenous Lines

Mannequins developed for skills training and high-fidelity scenarios have rubber tubing in their arms that mimic veins and connect to external drainage bags. As these mannequins age, the rubber tubing becomes fragile and requires replacement, which is not easy to do. Peripheral and central lines that do not use the internal rubber tubing system and are completely external are easy to set up and require no maintenance. The following sections include equipment lists and directions for setting up intravenous lines.

Triple Lumen Catheter

Equipment List

- Triple lumen catheter
- Large Tegaderm
- 14 Fr red rubber catheter
- Simulated BioPatch
- Fingernail polish (any color)
- Three needle free vales (SmartSites pictured) with flush
- Urinary drainage bag

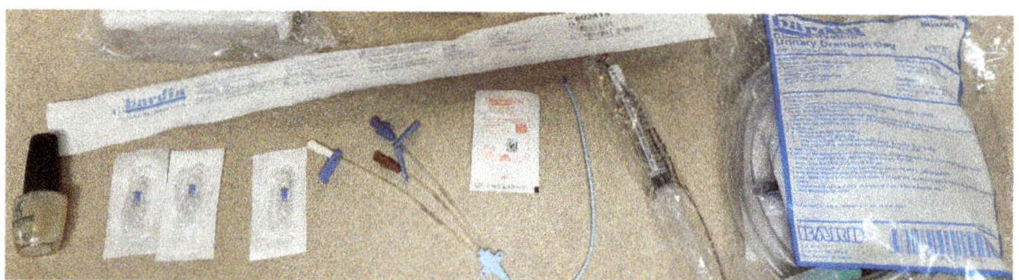

FIGURE 7.1 Supplies Needed for Triple Lumen Catheter

1. Open the red rubber catheter and cut the tip off, removing the open hole.
2. Insert triple lumen catheter until ALL its holes are within the red rub catheter.

3. Paint juncture of 2 catheters with a lot of nail polish. Let dry and repeat the process. Let it dry before use. This will seal the juncture, and no leaks will occur.

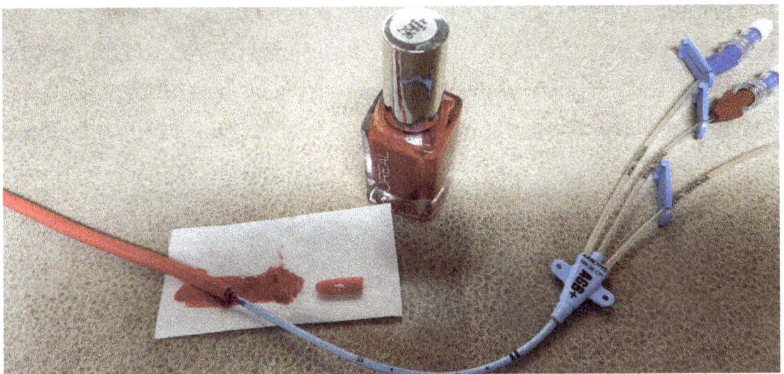

FIGURE 7.2 Application of Nail Polish to Seal Triple Lumen to Red Rubber Catheter

4. Place a needleless valve into each of the 3 ends of triple lumen catheter.
5. If the mannequin has openings, as shown in Figure 7.3, thread the red rubber catheter through the holes, then connect it to the urinary drainage bag.

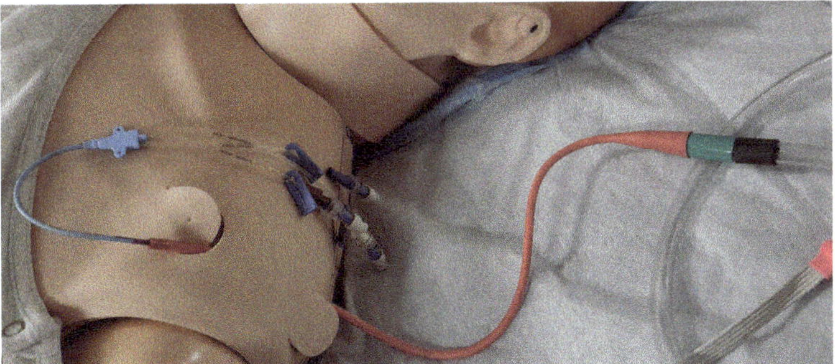

FIGURE 7.3 Triple Lumen Catheter Threaded Through Hole in Mannequin Chest and Attached to Drainage System

If you do not have mannequins with soft chest plates and slits already in place, you can make your own. Use a piece of an old mannequin chest or an old IV arm skin. Cut a square about 4" by 4" and cut a slit in it. Place it on the chest and thread the triple lumen catheter connected to the red rubber catheter through it and then connect the red rubber catheter to the urinary drainage bag. Place a simulated BioPatch around the catheter site and cover with a central dressing kit Tegaderm or any large Tegaderm. Cover the red rubber catheter with a chux to hide the magic.

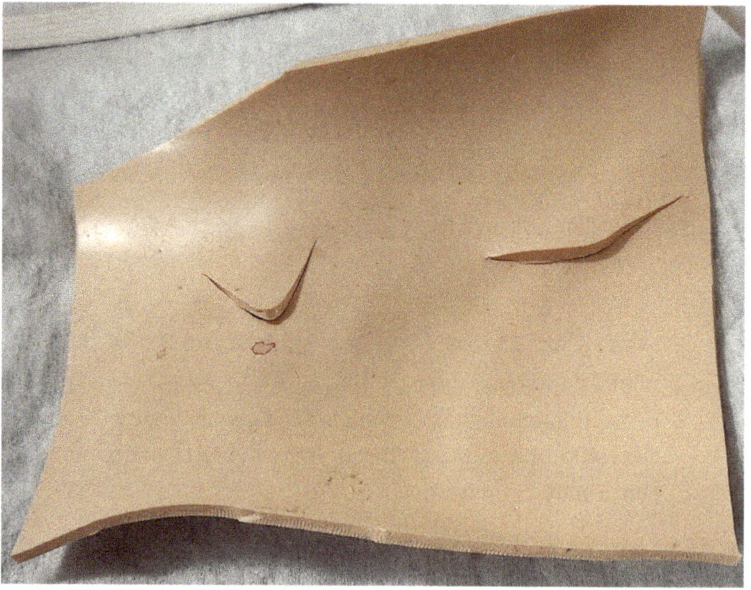

FIGURE 7.4 Piece of Soft Mannequin Skin with Slits Added to Use With Central Line Magic

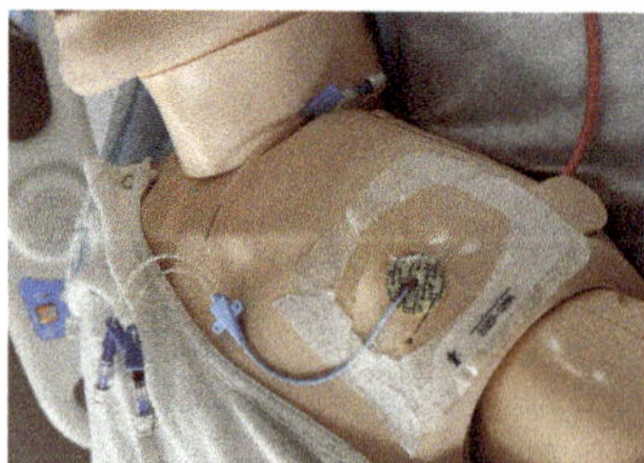

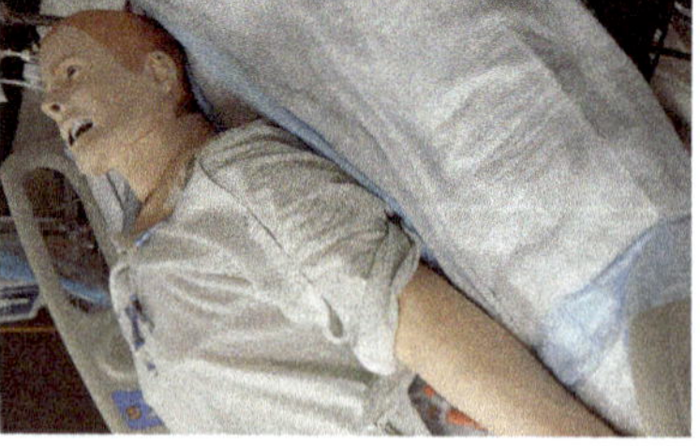

FIGURE 7.5 Triple Lumen With Simulated BioPatch and Tegaderm Dressing, Drainage System Covered With Chux

Peripheral Intravenous Lines

This system is a closed loop between the primary bag of IV fluids and the empty IV bag for drainage, with all tubing on the outside of the body and no needle in the system.

Equipment List

- Primary bag of IV fluids that are to be infused, spiked, and primed with whatever tubing is appropriate for infusion
- IV extension set
- Empty 1,000 mL IV bag
- Secondary IV tubing
- Small Tegaderm dressing
- 3-way stopcock OR female/female connector
- Coban wrap

1. Hang the primed bag of fluids and connect the end to the IV extension set and prime the extension tubing.
2. Position the middle of the extension tubing to where the IV site would be.
3. Place a small Tegaderm dressing over the spot in the extension tubing.
4. (The drainage system for peripheral IV fluids requires IV secondary tubing because it does not have valves in it and fluid will flow through it backward toward the empty drainage bag.) Spike the empty IV bag with the secondary tubing.
5. Connect the secondary tubing to a female site of the 3-way stopcock or to a female/female connector.
6. Connect the end of the extension tubing to either the second female site of the stopcock (A) or the open female connector site (B). (This gives you a closed loop from IV fluid bag to the empty drainage bag.)
7. Run the tubing up the arm and hang the empty bag beneath the head of the bed. Use the Coban to hide the magic, wrapping from the middle of the small Tegaderm dressing to the armpit.

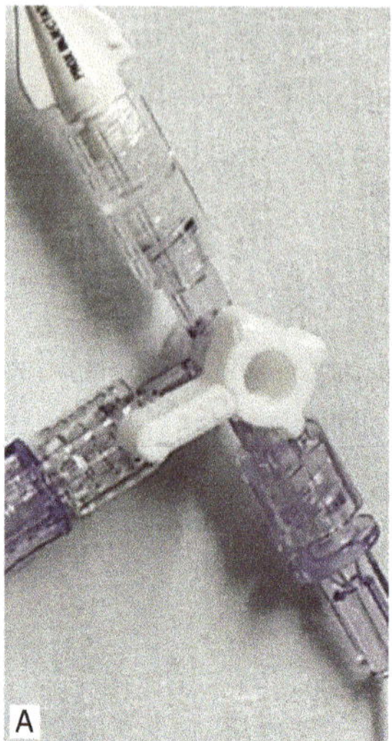

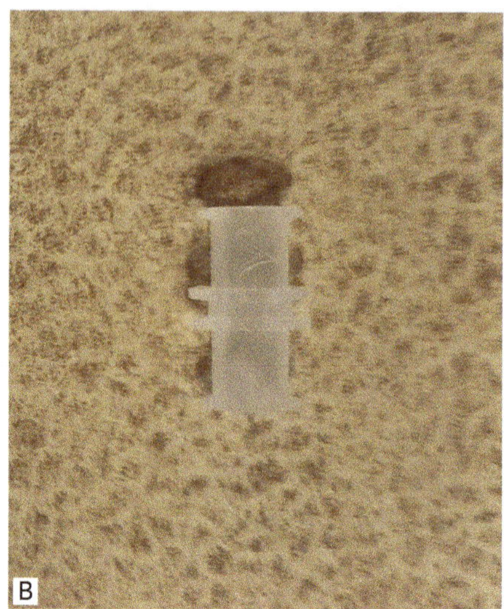

FIGURE 7.6 Where to Connect the Extension Tubing and the Secondary Tubing

Introducer Sheath

Introducer sheaths are necessary to float pulmonary catheters in position within the right side of the heart. They are essentially single lumen central lines.

Equipment List

- Percutaneous Sheath Introducer Kit (sometimes called a "Cordis" because they were the first manufacturer) or just the introducer sheath
- Red rubber catheter, usually 14 gauge
- Nail polish
- Urinary drainage bag
- Pulmonary artery catheter (PAC; generic) or Swan Ganz Catheter (optional, but if you want pulmonary artery pressures, you will need it; if you just want a central line, you just need the introducer sheath)
  - Plastic sheath that fits over catheter (condom catheter)
- Large Tegaderm for dressing

1. Open the red rubber catheter package and cut the tip off

2. If you are inserting a PAC through the introducer sheath, open it and the yellow plastic "condom sheath" that goes over the PAC.
3. Thread the end of the PAC through the bottom of the condom sheath.
4. Once it is on the PAC, thread the PAC into the introducer sheath where the black circle is and straight through the long white plastic sheath. Keep inserting it until all of the holes on the PAC are through the white sheath.
5. Take the PAC tip and thread it through the red rubber catheter until all of the yellow and half of the white sheath are within the red rubber catheter.
6. Apply the fingernail polish where the red rubber catheter and the white introducer sheath meet (several coats).

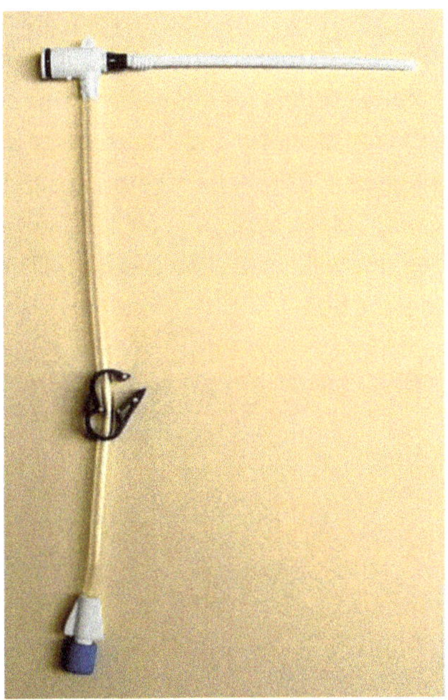

FIGURE 7.7 Introducer sheath, black circle at top left, insert yellow end of PAC into the black circle and straight down the long white tube until all the wholes are through it and some of the white sheath

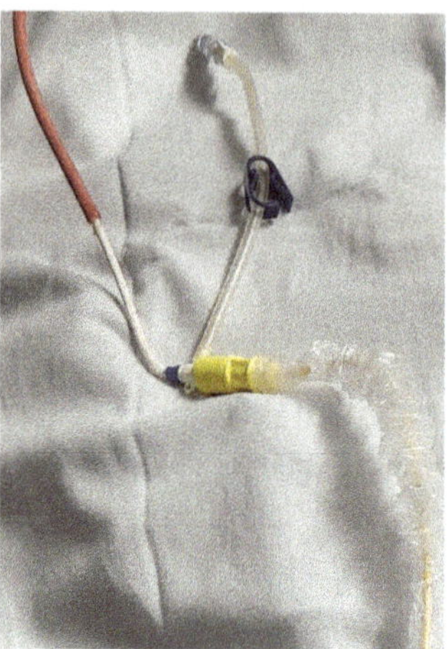

FIGURE 7.8 Once yellow catheter is positioned correctly through the white then red rubber tubes, add nail polish to white/red connection

Thread the red rubber catheter through the holes in the mannequin chest. There are many options for connecting this catheter to drainage. You can use the red catheter and connect it to a urinary drainage bag, but you might need a 16 French catheter, depending on the size of the introducer sheath. Make sure you can see the yellow PAC in your drainage tubing, as this will ensure the system will not leak. Hang the drainage bag below the bed.

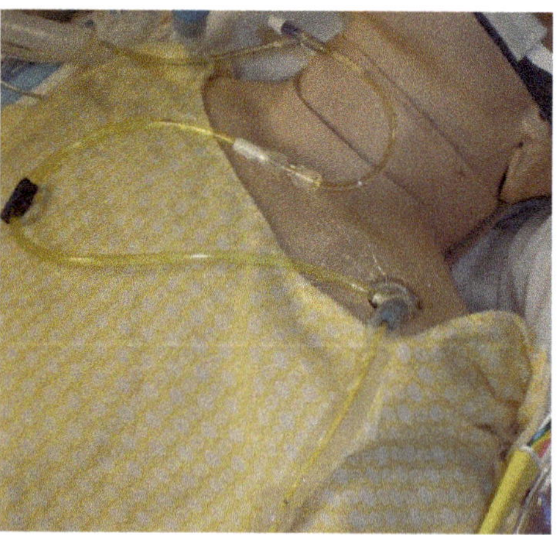

FIGURE 7.9 PAC Threaded Through Holes in Chest and Insertion Site Dressed With Large Tegaderm

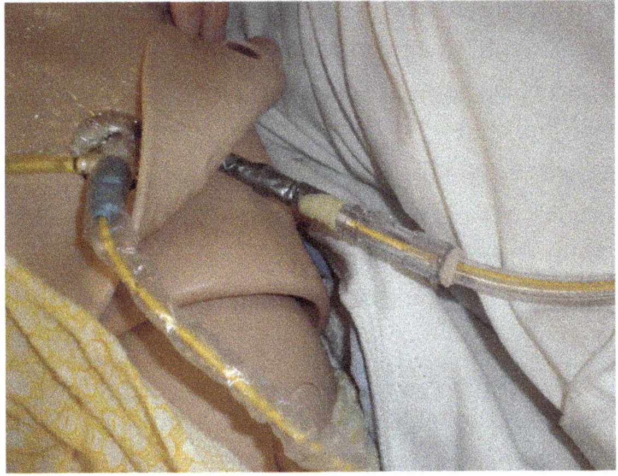

FIGURE 7.10 Chest Tube Used Instead of a Red Rubber Catheter and Then Connected to a Urinary Bag

Arterial Lines

Equipment List

- 500 mL bag of 0.9% sodium chloride
- Pressure bag
- Arterial line tubing and transducer
  - Keep in mind, arterial tubing has tubing that runs to a transducer, then a stopcock and a 6-inch piece of tubing that connects to an arterial catheter. This setup has a closed loop of arterial on one side of the arm and the blood for drawing arterial blood on the other side

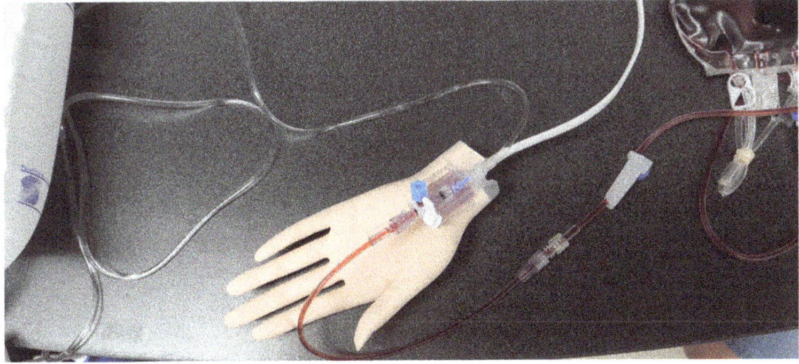

FIGURE 7.11 Arterial Line That Can Have Blood Drawn in Simulation

- Bag of blood spiked with secondary IV tubing
- Extension tubing with one end male and the other end female if not part of the arterial tubing setup
- Coban and chux
    1. Spike the sodium chloride with the arterial line tubing and place it in a pressure bag.
    2. Prime the arterial tubing.
    3. Spike the blood with the secondary tubing and add the extension tubing.
    4. Prime with blood.
    5. Connect the male ending of the arterial line tubing to the female ending of the extension tubing full of blood. This creates a closed loop. It allows blood to be drawn out of the stopcock on the arterial side of the tubing and then flushed back into the blood tubing to clear the line.
    6. Clamps on the sodium chloride bag side and the blood side must be open during simulation, or the arterial line won't work.

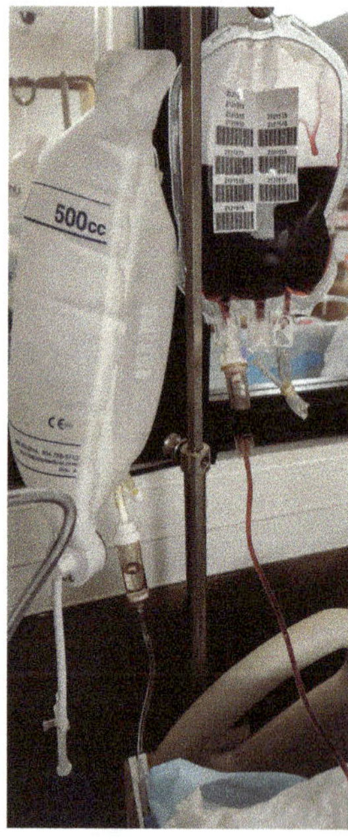

FIGURE 7.12 Arterial line hangs as is normal and blood bag supplies lab draws. Don't forget to place a bag or pillowcase over bag of blood and wrap arm

Percutaneous Esophagogastrostomy (PEG) Tubes

PEGs are inserted into all mannequins. This allows all oral medications to be given realistically, and allows students to make medication dosage calculations.

Equipment List

- PEG tubes with Lopez Valve
- Large urinary drainage catheter cut in half
- Urinary drainage bag
- Fingernail polish

Insert PEG into the half of the urinary drainage catheter that is connected to the urinary drainage bag. Use fingernail polish (several coats) to seal them together. Make sure when you cut the big urinary catheter (sizes 18–22) you throw away the part with the holes and balloon. Thread the PEG through any hole in the left side of the mannequin (some have flaps for chest tubes that you can put PEG through). Use multiple coats of nail polish to keep these tubes together. Dress the PEG site according to local hospital protocol.

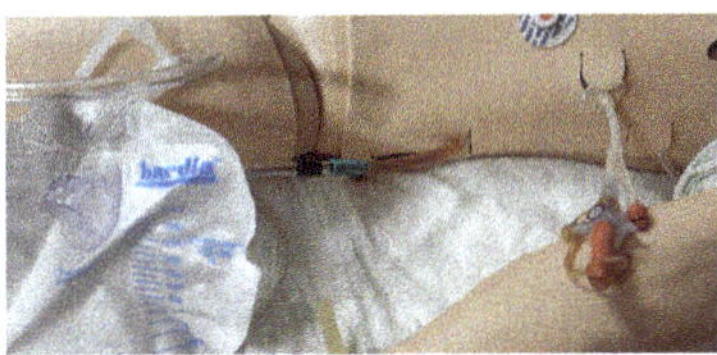

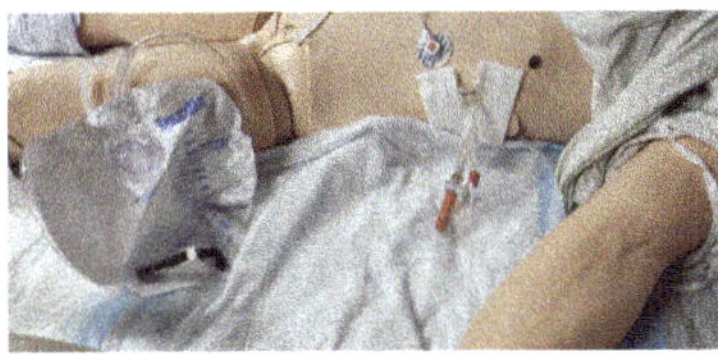

FIGURE 7.13 You can buy simulated PEG tubes from simulation stores

It is important that students learn to use evidence in administering tube feedings and medications via enteral feeding tubes. Below are the guidelines for administering medications via feeding tubes. These guidelines were published in 2009, and they are still state of the art. The only changes that are important regard the increase in medications that are released over time. These types of medications should not be given via enteral tubes. Crushing them alters their bioavailability with documented patient side effects.

ENTERAL NUTRITION AND MEDICATION ADMINISTRATION GUIDELINES

U.S. Department of Health & Human Services
AHRQ Agency for Healthcare Research and Quality
National Guideline Clearinghouse Guideline Summary
NCG-7288
Date Released: January 2009

Major Recommendations

Definitions of the grades of recommendations (**A-C**) are provided at the end of the "Major Recommendations" field.

Practice Recommendations

1. Do not add medication directly to an enteral feeding formula. **(B)**
2. Avoid mixing together medications intended for administration through an enteral feeding tube given the risks for physical and chemical incompatibilities, tube obstruction, and altered therapeutic drug responses (i.e., do not mix medications together, but do dilute them appropriately prior to administration). **(B)**
3. Each medication should be administered separately through an appropriate access. Liquid dosage forms should be used when available and if appropriate. Only immediate-release solid dosage forms may be substituted. Grind simple compressed tablets to a fine powder and mix with sterile water. Open hard gelatin capsules and mix powder with sterile water. **(B)**
4. Prior to administering medication, stop the feeding and flush the tube with at least 15 mL water. Dilute the solid or liquid medication as appropriate and administer using a clean oral syringe (> 30 mL in size). Flush the tube again with at least 15 mL water taking into account person's volume status. Repeat with the next medication (if appropriate). Flush the tube one final time with at least 15 mL

U.S. Department of Health and Human Services, Selection from "Eternal Nutrition and Medication Administration Guidelines," *Enteral Nutrition and Medication Administration Guidelines*, 2009.

water. Note: Dilution/flush should be less for pediatric doses (minimum 50:50 volume) and at least 5 mL when fluid is not restricted. **(A)**

5. Restart the feeding in a timely manner to avoid compromising nutrition status. Only hold the feeding by 30 minutes or more when separation is indicated to avoid altered drug bioavailability. **(A)**
6. Use only oral/enteral syringes labeled with "for oral use only" to measure and administer medication through an enteral feeding tube. **(B)**
7. Consult with a pharmacist for individuals who receive medications co-administered with enteral nutrition. **(C)**

Definitions: Grade of Recommendation

A. There is good research-based evidence to support the guideline (prospective, randomized trials).

B. There is fair research-based evidence to support the guideline (well-designed studies without randomization).

C. The guideline is based on expert opinion and editorial consensus.

Bibliographic Source(s)

Bankhead, R., Boullata, J., Brantley, S., Corkins, M., Guenter, P., Krenitsky, J., Lyman, B., Metheny, N. A., Mueller, C., Robbins, S., & Wessel, J. (2009). Enteral nutrition practice recommendations. *Journal of Parenteral Enteral Nutrition, 33*(2), 158–162.

Mannequins That Speak

Inexpensive walkie-talkies can allow the patients to answer questions by placing a walkie-talkie under their pillow.

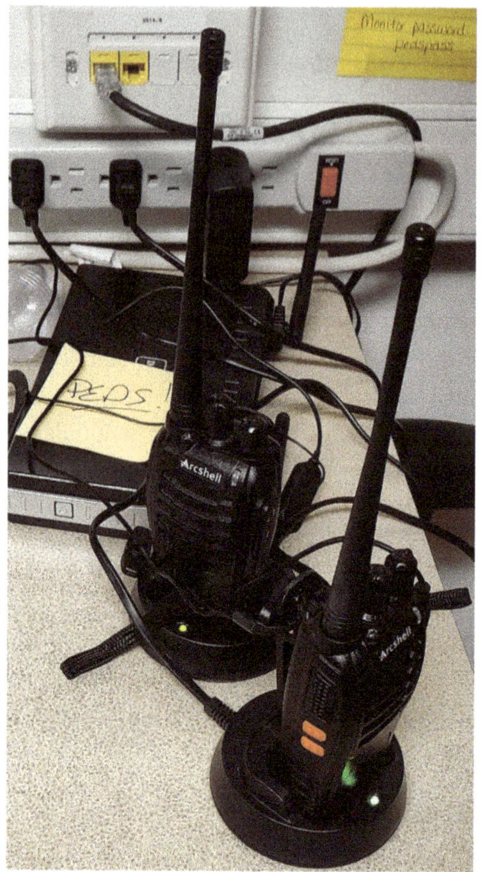

FIGURE 7.14 Walkie-Talkies to Enable Students to Ask Patients Questions

Important Tips

#1 Mannequin Skin and Tape

Mannequins skin does not like tape of any kind. It will eventually melt and make a sticky mess. Get large pieces of Tegaderm (8x12) and cut them into large strips and use them instead of tape. The Tegaderm pieces are invisible, they do not melt, and they stick nicely. (If you get expired equipment from the OR, be sure and get their dressing supplies, as they have very large pieces of Tegaderm.)

#2 Blood Sugar

To make fake blood that reads as blood sugar in a glucometer, you will need red food coloring, water, and a liquid form of glucose. Glucose can be found in grocery/department/drug stores that handle diabetic supplies. It needs to be liquid without flavors. You mix up batches in small bottles and track how many mL of colored water and how many mL or drops of glucose, then test the solution using a glucometer. Cut a finger off the glove, put cotton in the tip of the finger, add the glucose solution, and put the finger with the cotton glucose solution over the mannequin's finger. Put a rubber band on the finger to hold the gloved finger tightly in place. Stick the finger to get a blood drop on the glucometer to see what the blood sugar reads. This will give you a solution in low, normal, and high glucose readings as you experiment on your mixtures. There are also simulation companies that market blood glucose solutions and fake finger coverings. These are easier to use but much more expensive.

Summary

Nurses are very inventive when it comes to making reality for simulation. There are now multiple simulation stores online where you can buy simulated equipment, so sometimes it is worth the time to shop around for the best price. If you do the majority of your shopping at one particular simulation store, you can possibly get a deal with them that gives you a percentage of the price off for all of your purchases. It's worth exploring. When you purchase IV Pumps you need to decide if you need a maintenance package if you do not have biomed available to your school. You will also need to determine if you need a warranty on the mannequins as they are very expensive.

There are numerous simulation sites and books that offer tips on how to create the reality of simulation. All simulation conferences have exhibition halls where simulation mannequins and equipment are displayed. They frequently offer deals to people purchasing equipment and supplies at the conference.

Conclusion

This book tells the story of how to create a program of simulation that incorporates CJMM with a plan of student assessment that provides longitudinal data. The theory of deliberate practice provides the methodology for ensuring student mastery of psychomotor skills when a fundamentals class becomes a simulation experience. Mapping out the cognitive functions of CJMM within simulation scenarios allows for development of specific student performance behaviors in addition to calculating percent of successful completion of the behaviors. Change should always be data driven. The data derived from this program is relevant to student, course, and program outcomes.

Index

www.ingramcontent.com/pod-product-compliance
Ingram Content Group UK Ltd.
Pitfield, Milton Keynes, MK11 3LW, UK
UKHW021830270726
14058UKWH00001B/66

9 798823 320924